Office 365 for Healthcare Professionals

Improving Patient Care Through Collaboration, Compliance, and Productivity

Nidhish Dhru

Apress®

Office 365 for Healthcare Professionals

Nidhish Dhru
San Ramon, California, USA

ISBN-13 (pbk): 978-1-4842-3548-5   ISBN-13 (electronic): 978-1-4842-3549-2
https://doi.org/10.1007/978-1-4842-3549-2

Library of Congress Control Number: 2018940276

Managing Director: Welmoed Spahr
Acquisitions Editor: Joan Murray
Development Editor: Laura Berendson
Coordinating Editor: Jill Balzano

Cover designed by eStudioCalamar
Cover image designed by Freepik (www.freepik.com)

Distributed to the book trade worldwide by Springer Science+Business Media New York, 233 Spring Street, 6th Floor, New York, NY 10013. Phone 1-800-SPRINGER, fax (201) 348-4505, email orders-ny@springer-sbm.com, or visit www.springeronline.com. Apress Media, LLC is a California LLC and the sole member (owner) is Springer Science + Business Media Finance Inc (SSBM Finance Inc). SSBM Finance Inc is a **Delaware** corporation.

For information on translations, please email rights@apress.com, or visit http://www.apress.com/rights-permissions.

Apress titles may be purchased in bulk for academic, corporate, or promotional use. eBook versions and licenses are also available for most titles. For more information, reference our Print and eBook Bulk Sales web page at http://www.apress.com/bulk-sales.

Any source code or other supplementary material referenced by the author in this book is available to readers on GitHub via the book's product page, located at www.apress.com/9781484235485. For more detailed information, please visit http://www.apress.com/source-code.

Printed on acid-free paper

In July 2016, my family and I went through a very rough time due to my hospitalization over several weeks and recovery over several months. While lying in that hospital bed, I witnessed how things worked at the hospital, and I decided right then that I would write about improving productivity and collaboration between hospital staff and patients. This book will focus on that core idea of how to leverage tools that most healthcare providers have already invested in and put them to work to improve internal and external productivity and collaboration.

This book is for the healthcare professionals who are still skeptical about the cloud and its future. During my recent years of working with healthcare professionals I have seen a hesitation toward the change because of regulations and a concern about losing control over patient data. Hopefully this book will help you understand why the cloud is even more secure than existing data centers and how you can maximize your investments without worrying about downtime or continuous patching and maintenance headaches. The objective of this book is to help IT and business staff focus on what they do best, which is serving the patient and improving their health, instead of worrying about data centers, compliance, or security. My hope is that with the help of this book, IT will be able to focus more on adding value to business and in turn help improve patient care.

Table of Contents

About the Author

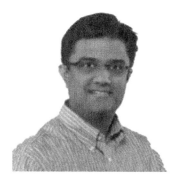 **Nidhish Dhru** is a husband, father, son, cloud strategist, and, most importantly, a lifelong learner. Nidhish has spent over 12 years working with several units within Microsoft and over 8 years with other systems integrators across various countries, such as India, Malaysia, Singapore, and now in the United States. Nidhish pursued his master's degree while working at Microsoft and enjoys all its learnings throughout the course of the business.

Nidhish is a problem solver who has helped many customers across the globe overcome their business challenges with creative ideas and exceptional technical guidance. Most recently, Nidhish has been involved with helping large enterprise customers transition to the cloud, specifically Office 365 and Azure. He specializes in and is most passionate about working with healthcare organizations to modernize their infrastructure, reducing operational costs and helping increase patient care via technology innovation. Nidhish presents at Microsoft Ignite and the Bay Area Healthcare Innovation Summit.

About the Technical Reviewer

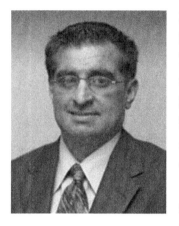

Dr. Sundeep Desai is the vice president and chief health information officer of the Valley Operating Unit of Sutter Health. He led the implementation of the electronic health record in both the ambulatory space and in the ten hospitals in his area over the last decade, and his responsibilities now include supporting the technology needs of the physicians throughout the Valley, with a focus on how to get the most value out of these technology investments.

He received his bachelor's degree and medical degree from the University of Michigan. He then completed an internal medicine residency at Northwestern University in Chicago, IL. He stayed there on the faculty of Northwestern University Medical School for eight years prior to coming to Sutter.

Acknowledgments

This book wouldn't have been possible without the learnings gleaned over years of implementing solutions for my customers in the healthcare space. I recently worked with the second-largest healthcare provider in Northern California and learned more than I contributed to their success. I was never an outsider, and they shared every detail of their healthcare environment, which allowed me and my team to help them find the right implementation of Office 365 services. My team presented at Microsoft's biggest customer event in Florida in September 2017 on the best practices to follow when implementing Office 365 in healthcare environments, which was received well, with very positive feedback. I want to acknowledge all those customers and colleagues I have had the good fortune to work with and thank them for their continuous mentorship and partnership.

My biggest inspiration for writing this book is my son, Tanishk. He wants to write a book full of characters with imaginary wars, like in *Star Wars*. While I agree that this book is not on par with Tanishk's stories, I promise I gave my best in writing it. I want to thank my wife, Sonali, for sticking with me during yet another challenge of writing a book that demanded more time away from family. She managed it all well and never made me feel what a bozo I am.

Finally, I want to thank Microsoft for providing a platform via which many individuals like me have achieved our dreams in the field of information technology. Microsoft has taught me patience, fellowship, leadership, and, more importantly, giving back to community. All these learnings came to the rescue while writing this book, and I hope you all enjoy reading it.

Introduction

The healthcare landscape is rapidly changing, and providers must improve and extend the care experience for patients by enabling greater productivity through modern, secure, and financially sustainable environments. Patients want access to providers in new ways, including faster communication and better transparency. Providers want to provide quality clinical-based care with a focus on operating efficiency and maximum patient satisfaction, thereby reducing lengths of stay and readmission rates and lowering costs. While every provider is unique, there are and will always be operational and clinical similarities between providers. This book will focus on sharing those best practices that can be applied to any healthcare provider that is willing to improve efficiency by transforming patient care.

This book will provide innovative ideas to those who are seeking higher productivity in healthcare. This book will help the reader understand why it is important to leverage the public cloud for healthcare and how to be more secure and more compliant with all healthcare compliance standards while still being more productive. This book will go through several topics, such as telehealth, readmission rate, nurse shift scheduling, tumor board innovations, continuous education for nurses and physicians, and so forth. Healthcare is a complex industry with ever more regulations, increasing costs, lower margins, longer innovation cycles, and a decreasing quality of care. This book will help readers realize that their existing investments in Office 365 can be maximized by demonstrating a completely different perspective that can result in cost reduction, faster innovation, and better patient care with tighter security and higher compliance standards.

This book will not talk about healthcare reforms at the national level nor share any perspective on what is wrong with the healthcare system. This book will focus on technological advancement via Office 365 in existing day-to-day operations in healthcare systems. This book has two specific goals for readers: first, increase the value of existing investments in Office 365 by leveraging its services more broadly outside of the IT organization, and second, solve real-time productivity and communication challenges by applying simple techniques via the existing toolset.

This book's innovative ideas will help providers

- be more efficient in both internal and external collaboration;

- reduce the cost of newer technology acquisition by utilizing existing investments;

- look at instant collaboration versus long and delayed conversations;

- improve tracking and logging of communication for detailed analysis; and

- improve patient satisfaction by bridging the communication gap.

CHAPTER 1

Improving Productivity in Healthcare with Office 365

Healthcare is a complex industry with ever more regulations, increasing costs, lower margins, longer innovation cycles, and decreasing quality of care. United States healthcare spending reached $3.2 trillion in 2015, accounting for 17.8 percent of the GDP. By the year 2021, it is projected to reach $4.8 trillion, accounting for one-fifth of the U.S. economy, according to the Center for Medicare and Medicaid Service (12/06/2016).[1] Despite this spending, the United States ranks behind most developed countries in various measures of health outcomes, such as affordability, accessibility, life expectancy, and healthcare costs per capita. Healthcare has become the top concern for Americans, even surpassing the economy, and rightly so. Wasteful practices play a major part in this problem, costing $750 billion dollars annually. A significant portion of these wasteful practices are the result of interoperability issues, which entail data-sharing challenges and communication gaps between different providers, hospitals, and payers. The information that is captured and tracked traditionally tends to stay only within a singular organization.

The healthcare industry has been traditionally slow to adopt innovative technology, such as the cloud, artificial intelligence (AI), Internet of Things, virtual reality, and so forth. These technological innovations loom on the health industry's horizon, with great potential to cause disruption in the next decade. These technologies are described in Figure 1-1.

---

[1] https://www.cms.gov/Research-Statistics-Data-and-Systems/Statistics-Trends-and-Reports/NationalHealthExpendData/NationalHealthAccountsHistorical.html

© Nidhish Dhru 2018
N. Dhru, *Office 365 for Healthcare Professionals*, https://doi.org/10.1007/978-1-4842-3549-2_1

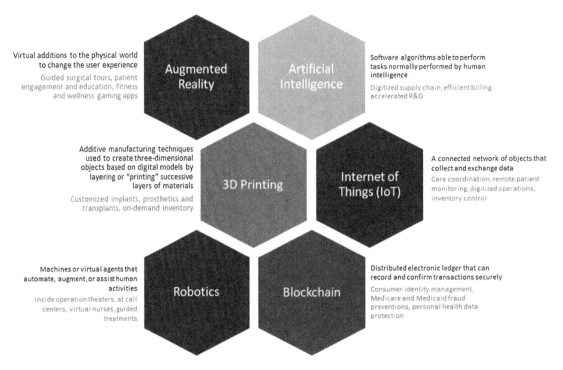

Figure 1-1. *Healthcare technology disruptors*

Traditionally, hospitals concentrated on taking care of patients while they were within the walls of the building. Today, there's a new model for healthcare, one in which hospitals and healthcare systems look beyond the facility itself, helping patients avoid hospital stays and ensuring the best possible long-term outcomes. That new model requires a new way of thinking about patients and how a healthcare system should operate to most efficiently care for them. Each of the preceding trends is going to disrupt healthcare for the next generation. While these innovations are happening, IT professionals need to decide whether to continue maintaining legacy systems or to help their line of business be more productive and innovative by adopting these disruptive technologies.

As just discussed, the healthcare landscape is rapidly changing, and providers must improve and extend the care experience for patients by enabling great productivity through modern, secure, and financially sustainable environments. Patients want access to providers in new ways, including faster communication and transparency. Providers want to provide quality clinical-based care with a focus on operating efficiency and maximum patient satisfaction, thereby reducing lengths of stay and keeping readmissions at a lower cost. While every provider is unique, there are and will always be operational and clinical similarities between providers. This book will focus on sharing best practices that can be applied to any healthcare provider that is willing to improve efficiency by transforming patient care.

In the following chapters, we will discuss innovative ideas for those who are seeking higher productivity in healthcare. We will explore why it is important to leverage the public cloud for healthcare and how to be more secure and more compliant with all healthcare compliance standards while still being more productive. We will review several topics, such as telehealth, readmission rates, nurse shift scheduling, tumor board innovations, continuous education for nurses and physicians, and so on. This book is designed to teach healthcare organizations how to increase the productivity of clinicians and information workers. It does so using real-world examples that serve as a guide to using Office 365 to support cost reduction, faster innovation, and better patient care with tighter security and higher compliance standards.

Need for Innovation

In recent years, the healthcare industry has been victimized by cyberattacks and new threat vectors, which has resulted in ramped up regulatory requirements and enforcement of these requirements. This has caused security to become a strategic business requirement for any healthcare provider. Security, which at one point was an afterthought, is now at the front and center of all innovations. Industry data shows the average healthcare breach costs $355 per record stolen and approximately $2.2 million per breach event. IT is faced with tremendous pressure to keep organizations safe and secure while offering open and collaborative solutions to line-of-business stakeholders. There is a need for evolution and advances in healthcare information technology that will drive innovative technical solutions and improve organizational efficiency, population health, and patient outcomes across the continuum of care.

The lack of collaboration capabilities in electronic health record (EHR) systems causes clinician inefficiencies and dissatisfaction. According to a recent IDC Health Insights survey, the top two reasons for physician job dissatisfaction were related to being less productive—either because more time was spent on documentation (85 percent) or because physicians were not able to see more patients (66 percent). Most EHRs do not follow physicians' workflows, and to overcome this disjointed experience many physicians are recommending that healthcare organizations invest in true unified communications and personal productivity tools to support effective clinician communication and collaboration.

Patient safety is at risk because of the lack of proper communication and information handoffs between shift changes. This results in redundant tests, miscommunication of patient health, and patient dissatisfaction. In fact, the Joint Commission Sentinel Event database reveals that poor communication is the root cause in nearly 70 percent of reported sentinel events, which it defines as unexpected events involving death or serious physical or psychological injury, or risk thereof, not related to the natural course of the patient's illness.

Physicians and nurses use multiple devices, such as laptops, workstations, tablets, and smartphones, in addition to shared workstations throughout their workday. Physicians and nurses demand a seamless continuation of their work no matter which device they are on at a given time. It is important to note that the security of the content is essential in order to avoid leaking patient health information (PHI). Healthcare providers need a platform that is not only secure but also highly portable. Such a platform should include the following:

- End-to-end encryption
- Privacy and security
- Regulatory compliance support
- Information security strategy and policies approach
- Mobile device management (MDM) options
- Data loss prevention (DLP) capabilities, rules, and policies
- Audit logging and monitoring configurations
- Access controls and permissions

One recent innovative example in the medical space is the digital pill. Most physicians cringe at the thought of their patient attempting to correctly take their complicated pill regimen without even being able to see the pills. With the help of technology, it can be a little easier to track if the patient is taking the right medication at the right time in the prescribed quantity. Recently, the FDA approved a digital pill that can tell the doctor if the patient is taking the medicine or not. The pill, called the Ability MyCite, is embedded with a sensor that tracks ingestion. The digital pill will first be used with schizophrenia and bipolar disorder patients, and could also be part of the treatment for depression. When ingested, the sensor registers against a smart patch worn by the patient, and it transmits data to a phone. In turn—if the patient chooses— that information can be shared with medics, caregivers, or family members. That could be particularly useful for elderly people with faltering memories, for example, to track whether they are taking their drugs. This technology will reduce the bill caused by non-adherence to prescriptions, which for the United States has been estimated at up to $100 billion per year. Based on the data, providers can either send the nurse to visit the patient or leverage social workers to visit the patient regularly to help them follow the proper regimen.[2]

Iowa-based UnityPoint Health, in another example of innovation, used big data and analytics to reduce the readmission rate. There is no use for data if there is no learning from it, and that is what UnityPoint Health did by putting analytics to work on data they gathered over many years. With a keen focus on encouraging a culture that embraces the value of data and stays attuned to the unique needs of various stakeholders, the health system managed to achieve a 40 percent reduction in its risk-adjusted readmission index over three years at a pilot hospital.[3]

Office 365 Overview

Healthcare organizations are recognizing the economic and team-collaboration advantages of cloud computing and are overcoming what were once deep-seated concerns that the cloud, especially the public cloud, was not secure enough for healthcare. Taking an incremental approach to the cloud, many healthcare organizations are now selectively migrating operational workloads to the cloud before moving mission-critical clinical applications. Collaborative applications are top candidates for this migration strategy; 21.4 percent of provider IT executives reported that they were currently delivering or planned to deliver collaborative applications via a cloud solution.[4]

Healthcare organizations ranging from providers and payers to business associates have looked in recent years to take advantage of cloud-hosted platforms like Microsoft's Office 365 solution to drive efficiency and boost productivity amidst growing resource and budget constraints. This book outlines key considerations and leading practices for securely deploying Office 365 in a healthcare setting. Office 365 is a robust platform with

---

[2]November 13, 2017; https://www.fda.gov/NewsEvents/Newsroom/PressAnnouncements/ucm584933.htm

[3]Mike Miliard, August 23, 2017, 3:20 PM from Healthcare IT News, www.healthcareitnews.com

[4]IDC's Global Technology and Industry Research Organization IT Survey

a variety of capabilities and security features. The recommendations provided in this book should be leveraged to take advantage of the lessons learned from other healthcare entities that have worked to optimize the security and compliance of their Office 365 deployments.

Evolving employee and patient expectations that they be able to access the services and information they need faster and in a much more personalized manner mean a highly connected workplace, the new differentiator for quality care. Highly connected health organizations deliver secure information sharing and collaboration in real time, which can dramatically reduce costs and maximize resources. With Office 365, health professionals can easily work together within and across departments, agencies, and organizations with anywhere, multi-device access to email, web conferencing, patient records, and calendars. Furthermore, Office 365 is designed to meet healthcare-specific requirements for patient-centered collaboration, robust security, and adherence to privacy regulations such as HIPAA, ISO 27001, and EU Model Clauses.

Many healthcare providers have already started adopting cloud infrastructure to avoid costly on-premises solutions such as Active Directory and Exchange Server to reap the benefits of the cloud, such as scalability, ease of access, and low maintenance. The Office 365 platform includes Office products like Word, Excel, PowerPoint, Outlook, OneNote, and so on, messaging services such as instant messaging and online meetings (Skype), TEAMS, Exchange Online, and so forth, cloud file storage via OneDrive for Business, and collaboration via SharePoint Online. Microsoft recently introduced new applications, such as Power Apps, Flow, Planner, Sway, and Stream. Planner provides team collaboration and helps to organize work and assign tasks. Sway provides interactive digital storytelling and represents a step up from traditional PowerPoint-based presentation models. Power Apps provides drag-and-drop functionality to create line of business (LOB) apps with many connectors. Flow automates the process across LOB applications via an easy-to-configure workflow and connectors. Stream provides an enterprise video portal for video streaming with high fidelity. We will talk about each of these products via real-life use cases in subsequent chapters.

Office 365 Benefits for Healthcare Organizations

In this section, we will observe the benefits of using Office 365 in any healthcare environment. Figure 1-2 shows different benefits of using Office 365 in a healthcare environment.

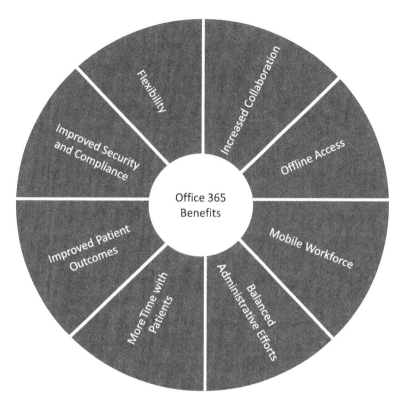

Figure 1-2. *Benefits of using Office 365 in healthcare*

Increased Collaboration

Office 365 allows you to connect with your colleagues in real time, allowing physicians and nurses to be more productive without losing time searching for people on the hospital floors or in clinics. Skype for Business, Outlook, SharePoint, OneDrive for Business, MS Teams, and Yammer give a clear indication of someone's presence via green, red, and yellow icons. Users can tap that person right from Skype for Business or Yammer and involve them in conversations via either instant messaging or voice/video calls. Tools like these in Office 365 can transform how people work and how the organization operates. Many healthcare organizations have various locations between which traditional collaboration and coordination were very difficult. With Office 365 and its collaboration tools, it is easy for people in all roles to collaborate at any place using any device.

For example, patient transfer from one department to another is a common workflow in healthcare. A nurse from the ER must call the ICU to contact the ICU nurse in order to give them the report of the patient that is about to be transferred to them.

This makes it take longer than necessary to move a patient from one department to another. By leveraging Skype for Business, using presence indicators to find out if the ICU nurse is there or not, and then quickly instant messaging or voice/video calling that nurse in the ICU, the ER nurse can expedite the entire process. Every minute saved in this process can result in improved patient care and better health outcomes.

Another important fact to note from a collaboration perspective is that having easy access to information, such as standard of care best practices, being able to communicate and consult in real time with other patient caregivers, and reducing travel around the hospital at any time during the workday for any clinician or physician are added advantages that improve patient care and its outcomes. SharePoint Online, OneDrive for Business, and Skype for Business help in making that information available in real time so that clinical workers spend more time on patient care and less time on administrative activities. Having access to the necessary information enables associates to make better decisions.

SharePoint Online can be used to survey patient satisfaction while patients are in the hospital, adjust the environment, or coach caregivers so that patients can heal faster. This information helps ensure that the right resources are at the right hospital with the right patient. Changes in nursing policies or procedures can be made available in real time so that patient care can be improved. Having a centralized location for all the documents helps save time and reduce the rework and errors when synthesizing feedback from multiple people. Simultaneous editing of documents can help doctors and nurses work on the same document from different locations, saving time that would have been spent emailing the same document multiple times and reducing concerns that information might get lost in multiple versions. Physicians sitting in the ICU can improve the relationship with the patient's relatives or with other clinicians by leveraging Skype for Business via face-to-face consultations. It helps staff make decisions faster, reduces costs, and gets patients out of the ICU faster.

Enterprise social networking tools such as Yammer, part of Office 365, can be used companywide to make critical announcements or to start an initiative. A hospital at one location can start a Yammer group on how they are better serving their patients so that other facilities can learn and contribute to that best practice. Hospitals can also broadcast outbreaks of a disease at a certain location so that other hospitals can get prepared and serve their patients appropriately. Yammer is a social enterprise application that helps to break down company barriers to connect people and information and enable better decisions, faster. As of November 2015, Yammer is covered as part of the standard HIPAA BAA for Microsoft Enterprise Online Services with Office 365. This makes Yammer a compliant solution for those health organizations wanting to connect all employees to share learning, collaborate, and act quickly to improve patient care and employee productivity. Yammer helps make the most of your network, offering you the ability to navigate, discover, and search across the organization to stay connected to the topics that matter most.

Office 365 also provides video portals where information workers such as IT staff, training team members, or clinical people from various organizational units can upload professionally created videos and share them with the broader organization. These videos are easily searchable via enterprise search, with a dedicated search experience in the video portal already scoped to show only video results. Video portals can be used for online training via any device from any location. This helps clinicians and physicians to view training material at their convenience and always be up-to-date with the information that can help improve patient care and experience.

Office 365 comes with Planner, a simple and highly visual way to organize teamwork. Planner makes it easy for teams to create new plans, organize and assign tasks, share files, chat about what they're working on, and get updates on progress. Planner is a lightweight project-management tool that can be used for smaller, less complex projects. Through Planner, you can be confident that you are making informed decisions that are right for you and your patients today and into the future. Planner helps reduce wait times by optimizing bed planning, appointment allocation, and overall capacity utilization. Planner helps in optimizing the utilization of facilities including wards, theaters, and treatment rooms to increase productivity. Planner ensures that you comply with all relevant working-time directives and minimize the occurrence of overtime and undertime payments.

Be Productive Without Internet

Does your organization have a requirement to keep information at one place and reuse it no matter where the user is and which device they are using, with or without internet? Physicians are asking to have information available to them all the time, with or without internet, using any device. In that scenario, having offline copies of data and syncing back while online helps. Office 365 offers offline editing capabilities from its rich client apps, which helps ensure version control is no longer a concern. Resolving conflicting changes is a feature enabled on files stored, shared, and worked on from OneDrive for Business (online or offline). This capability helps users know exactly what final version is being saved for future use. Offline copies of files help physicians to review the case and update the comments while not connected to internet. Once connected to the internet, changes are automatically synced to the document library in OneDrive or SharePoint.

Again, Office 365 makes sure that critical information is not lost, which can happen when maintaining separate versions of the same file in different locations. Information or clinical workers do not have specific setup requirements in order to collaborate with peers on offline documents.

Mobile Workforce

Does your organization have a need to help clinicians and information workers who are always on the go? Office 365 makes it easy for mobile workers to access their content securely and easily from any location via any device at any time. Office 365 apps such as Word/PowerPoint/Excel/OneNote, SharePoint, OneDrive, Planner, and Skype for Business are available on Windows, Android, and iOS devices. It is critical for healthcare organizations to have their workers be fully productive while on the go, even beyond traveling between different geographic locations. Nurses are always moving between patient rooms, taking notes, and calling on doctors for consultations either in person or via voice. Office 365 helps make nurses more productive as their work is stored securely in Office 365 and can be made available on both their handheld tablets and their workstations—no need to write notes on paper and then input them in the computer at a workstation!

Security is built into the apps mentioned. Without the right level of authentication and authorization, clinicians cannot get into any of the content. Via application-management policies, clinicians cannot copy/paste information from their corporate emails to personal emails, and cannot save corporate documents to their personal cloud storage, like OneDrive. All the content is stored encrypted inside those apps and on devices so that content is secure at rest. Multifactor authentication (MFA) is built into Office 365 services. MFA prompts for second-factor authentication, like a onetime PIN, password, phone authentication, and so forth, so that access to highly sensitive content is secure. This helps clinicians on the go have access to relevant files, calendars, emails, and SharePoint Online sites securely and quickly.

Office 365 mobile apps help nurses and physicians save time— as much as one hour a day in walking around the hospitals and two hours or more in visiting different facilities via virtual meetings, instant messaging, presence indicators, and one-on-one or one-to-many voice/video calls.[5] The Calendar app helps remind clinicians and physicians

---

[5]Business Value Realization with Office 365, A Total Economic Impact™ Analysis of Microsoft Office 365, A Forrester Total Economic Impact™ Study, March 2017

about important meetings and appointments so that patients don't have to wait long in hospital lobbies or waiting rooms.

Balanced Administrative Effort

On average, clinicians can save up to two hours a week on administrative activities as a result of having faster access to information and people and enjoying improved coordination across multiple departments and facilities.[6] This time can be spent on more valuable activities without increasing total hours worked, mainly spending more time with patients. Scheduling meetings, which used to take hours, can now be set up in minutes by looking at everyone's availability via shared calendars and by instant messaging them to check their availability. Automated task reminders and completion notifications can increase project-tracking accuracy in real time via SharePoint and Planner applications. Any information worker can look at someone else's free/busy calendar and book an appointment without needing to have admins look at everyone's availability manually.

Information workers and managers can now track how the organization is doing via Office 365 Workplace Analytics. Workplace Analytics provides rich, actionable insights into a company's communication and collaboration trends to help them make more effective business decisions. Microsoft Workplace Analytics analyzes how teams work together so that managers can identify the behaviors that help or hurt the bottom line. Workplace Analytics can help improve organizational efficiency, reduce job-related stress, reduce organizational chaos, engage and retain employees, gain insights into practice and provider performance, and bring data to life with easy-to-use dashboards and interactive reports.

Office 365 Delve Analytics can help individuals understand how they communicate and spend time at work. Workplace Analytics is at the organizational level and helps managers, whereas Delve Analytics is at the individual level and helps individuals make appropriate adjustments to their work style. Information workers can plan and exercise conscious control over the amount of time spent on specific activities, especially to increase effectiveness, efficiency, and productivity. Information workers or clinicians can set up their own work-related goals and let Delve Analytics measure their progress. For example, your average time in meetings as compared to the average time people in

---

[6]Page 4, Business Value Realization with Office 365, A Total Economic Impact™ Analysis of Microsoft Office 365, A Forrester Total Economic Impact™ Study, March 2017

your organization spend in meetings, or what percentage of the members of a group read a specific email. Delve Analytics empowers information workers or clinicians with the insights they need to work smarter and better balance their schedules by analyzing how other people use their time in the workplace and helping them manage their personal targets or organizational averages.

Less Time on the Road and More Time with Patients

Many knowledge workers, such as nurses and physicians, as well as clinical workers travel between facilities, from just a few miles away to a few cities away. Office 365 offers a robust virtual-meeting platform via Skype for Business to help facilities organize more online meetings to help reduce time spent traveling. IT, HR, nursing managers, and physicians can all benefit from this online voice or video conferencing. This not only saves time but also saves on transportation costs as well as reduces traveling stress. Skype for Business offers screen-sharing solutions where a nurse can share her/ his screen with a physician at a different location to get a consultation on a patient's condition or even see the patient remotely via Skype for Business video calls. This helps physicians provide expert opinions at the right time during the patient's treatment, which can improve the patient's health outcomes.

Skype for Business (SFB) helps staff communicate and collaborate from anywhere with HD-quality video streaming, desktop sharing, presenting, and more. SFB helps reach thousands while allowing meeting attendees to join from almost any browser or device. It simplifies conferencing management for both attendees and IT via a single vendor and support channel. SFB offers unified real-time enterprise communication services such as instant messaging, presence information, audio/web/ video conferencing, PSTN conferencing, desktop sharing, data sharing via electronic interactive whiteboards, call controls, integrated voicemail, email, SMS, and meetings. SFB enables meetings for small and large teams or up to 10,000 participants, who can join from any device anywhere. SFB also offers PSTN conferencing dial-in into meetings, Cloud PBX (a complete PBX replacement), and PSTN calling directly from Microsoft. SFB allows end-to-end security, compliance, and control—from the user to the enterprise— and is fully HIPAA compliant with a BAA.

Modern healthcare providers are constantly looking for innovative ways to service and connect to their patients and care teams. Microsoft recently announced the publication of new developer templates that extend Skype for Business as a platform for virtual healthcare. Office 365 with Skype for Business Online addresses the critical communication needs of healthcare providers, and these templates enable new mediums of care coordination for patients without requiring an Office 365 subscription. The Office 365 Virtual Health Templates allow you to accelerate building your virtual consult experiences by providing an open source solution using the Skype for Business SDKs announced earlier in 2016. These SDKs are powered by Office 365 and Skype for Business Online and support building web and mobile experiences that integrate presence, chat, audio, and video with custom business experiences. The templates use modern web-development technologies and leverage existing Skype for Business video services, making it easier for developers to build their own portals and apps that are integrated with other healthcare applications, like electronic health record (EHR) management systems and scheduling systems. Healthcare organizations can build telemedicine apps using Office 365 and Skype for Business (SFB) SDKs to support various telehealth programs. Hospitals can increase the number of patients they see in a day via SFB across all the programs.

Improved Patient Outcomes

An important thing for any healthcare provider is to improve patient outcomes and reduce readmission rates. With Office 365 and its services, providers can now focus more on patient care coordination and have better access to nonpatient information, such as patient satisfaction surveys, standards-of-care policies, and tracking of outcomes to improve patient care. Clinical workers save time by streamlining processes such as patient transfers and through improved access to all the information they needed regardless of location: patient room, nursing station, and so forth.

Does your organization have a requirement to minimize the amount of time clinical staff spends traveling to see patients, whether that's moving from hospital to hospital or from floor to floor? Skype for Business can facilitate multidisciplinary rounds, which in turn may reduce length of stay and readmissions, and may also improve patient satisfaction. Video calls via Skype for Business Online help multidisciplinary rounds for some hospitals' ICUs as well as for other facilities. Multidisciplinary rounds can take place by moving a wheeled workstation around each ICU so that all the caregivers involved can coordinate the patient's care without traveling from one hospital to another. Physicians can monitor patients using video from anywhere, take note of onscreen vital signs, and immediately provide consultation for course correction. This setup helps in situations where physicians cannot meet the patient in person but still have to diagnose the situation from a distance.

For healthcare providers, it is important that patients, after going home, follow the prescribed procedure to recover faster and avoid readmittance. Hospitals can leverage Office 365 and its services, such as SharePoint and SFB, to stay in touch with patients even after they go home. Clinicians or training members can upload how-to videos or create a list of frequently asked questions (FAQs) in SharePoint so that patients can stay well informed and can resolve their common questions. Systems like this help clinicians to be proactive in serving their patients better by helping in areas in which patients might have trouble managing their health.

Easier IT Security and HIPAA Compliance

Moving to Office 365 has made it easier and less expensive for providers to keep in place the necessary IT security, such as document and email security. Office 365 offers Advanced Threat Protection (ATP) to safeguard the email environment against potential threats. ATP protects organizations against zero-day malware attacks by making sure information workers and clinicians can only access links and email attachments that have been identified as not malicious.

Office 365 also made Health Insurance Portability and Accountability Act (HIPAA) compliance easier through better IT security and monitoring. More information on compliance and security is discussed in the following section.

Flexibility

Office 365 makes organizations more agile. Users can quickly move from one task to the next since they have easy access to all their information. Additionally, providers can more quickly launch new products and initiatives since employees can effectively collaborate. There are also additional opportunities and benefits that arise as new Office 365 features are launched. More and more features are getting rolled into the Office 365 platform without your even paying more, which increases the return on investment (ROI) in Office 365. One such example is the introduction of Microsoft TEAM. MS TEAM is one the most popular services in Office 365 and has been widely successful since its inception; it was included without any additional cost to existing customers. Providers can get the benefit of these new services as they roll out, and IT doesn't even have to buy any new infrastructure or spend money to deploy and configure them. Users can start using a new feature the day it is available in the Office 365 tenant. At the same time,

IT has full control over when to release the service to the end user based on user training or any regulatory compliance requirements. All the services in Office 365 are or will be HIPAA compliant, so IT doesn't have to do any additional work getting the service certified separately.

Meeting Security and Compliance Standards

Healthcare providers own and have full control of their data, even though it sits inside the Microsoft cloud. At any point if the healthcare organization decides to not use Office 365, they can take the data out of the Microsoft cloud. When you entrust your data to Office 365, you remain the sole owner of that data; you retain the rights, title, and interest in the data you store in Office 365. It's Microsoft's policy to not mine your data for advertising purposes or use your data except for purposes consistent with providing you cloud productivity services. Healthcare organizations can meet their needs by customizing the series of integrated security and compliance options. The following sections outline specific security and compliance capabilities, including encryption, regulatory compliance, DLP, audit logging and monitoring, access controls, and MDM integration. Office 365 ensures security and compliance by

- protecting data at rest via secure messaging with encryption;

- applying data loss prevention to content stored in Office 365 and reducing vulnerabilities;

- ensuring access controls are in place even if user is out of the corporate network via multi-factor authentication (MFA);

- providing quality patient care and security in environments of fragmented communication, information, and work processes;

- securing content inside mobile devices within and outside of corporate walls; and

- monitoring and logging every event possible for traceability to better serve as well as tackle user behaviors.

Figure 1-3 shows Office 365 security and compliance standards.

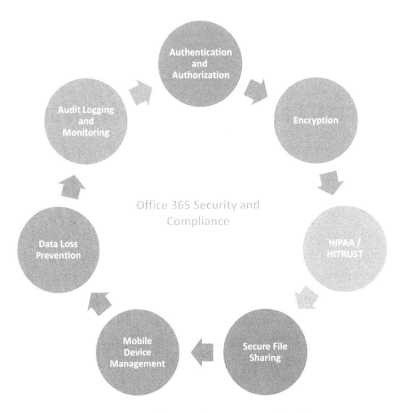

Figure 1-3. *Office 365 security and compliance standards*

Authentication and Authorization

Azure Active Directory is the backbone of Office 365 and is where it manages all the users. There are several options to manage user accounts and their access to Office 365, as follows:

- Cloud Identity: Users are created and managed in Azure Active Directory; user's corporate credentials are different from cloud credentials. These types of identities are good for quickly testing various services in Office 365.

- Synchronized Identity: Users are synchronized from on-premises directory to Azure Active Directory. Directory Synchronization tool is used for syncing users from on-premises Active Directory to Azure AD. User's passwords are synchronized across on-premises and cloud implementations.

- Federated Identity: Users are synchronized from on-premises directory to Azure Active Directory. Directory Synchronization tool is used for syncing users from on-premises Active Directory to Azure AD. User's passwords are *not* synchronized across on-premises and cloud implementations. Single sign-on (SSO) providers such as ADFS, Ping, Okta can be used to provide SSO between on-premises applications and Office 365.

- Role-Based Access Control (RBAC): Office 365 uses permission model to distribute different levels of permissions to different audiences. Administrators can create different roles and assign different permission levels. Users are then added to these roles for access to Office 365.

Encryption Options

Encryption is an important part of your file-protection and information-protection strategies. Office 365 provides end-to-end encryption for content both at rest and in transit. Encryption by itself does not prevent content—such as data, files, or email messages—from getting into the wrong hands. Encryption should be part of a larger information-protection strategy for any healthcare organization in order to protect highly sensitive data, including PHI. Encryption makes sure that only those who should be able to read encrypted content are able to.

Encryption for Data at Rest

Office 365 encrypts files stored in Office 365 data centers via BitLocker with AES 256-bit encryption. Files uploaded to SharePoint Online or OneDrive for Business, files updated in Skype for Business meetings, and email messages that are stored in folders are some examples of encrypted data at rest. Encryption is done by private key–value pair. Organizations can also bring their own key to encrypt the data so no one is able to look at the highly sensitive data without the customer's private key. However, this creates challenges in running the analytics tools offered by Office 365, as encryption prevents Office 365's services from reading the data and hence they cannot produce any analytical findings.

BitLocker volume encryption addresses the threats of data theft or exposure from lost, stolen, or inappropriately decommissioned computers and disks. Office 365 stores files uploaded in SharePoint or OneDrive for Business in separate databases with their own encryption keys. Those encryption keys are also encrypted and stored in a separate database with the encrypted map of file locations.

Encryption for Data in Transit

Office 365 encrypts all the incoming and outgoing traffic using TLS/SSL encryption. Internally in Office 365, server-to-server communication is also encrypted via TLS encryption. Email messages sent and received, conversations happening during online meetings, and documents being uploaded in SharePoint or OneDrive for Business are examples of data in transit. Emails and documents can also be rights protected using Rights Management Service, which uses AES 128-bit encryption keys, so that the content is appropriately used by specified people. Email encryption occurs by default and works behind the scenes so users don't have worry about encrypting or decrypting emails before sending or receiving them.

HIPAA (Health Insurance Portability and Accountability Act) with BAA

The Health Insurance Portability and Accountability Act (HIPAA) is a US healthcare law that establishes requirements for the use, disclosure, and safeguarding of individually identifiable health information. HIPAA regulations require that Office 365–covered entities and their business associates—in this case, Microsoft when it provides services, including cloud services, to covered entities—enter into contracts Business Assosicate Agreement (BAA) to ensure that those business associates will adequately protect patient health information (PHI).

The law regulates the use and dissemination of PHI in four general areas, as follows:

- Privacy: Patient information is the most critical and important information a healthcare provider has. Maintaining the privacy of that information is crucial, and Office 365 provides those compliance standards with HIPAA and a BAA.

- Security: Protection of information both physical and administrative to safeguard the healthcare information is paramount. Office 365 provides transparency for both the physical security of their data centers as well as administrative access to customers' data.

- Identifiers: The law prohibits the release of information collected for research purposes. Office 365 doesn't use any of this information for any advertising purposes and claims that the customer owns and controls their data.

- Codes are used for the electronic transmission of data in healthcare-related transactions, including eligibility and insurance claims and payments. Office 365 doesn't use customers' information for any advertising purpose and claims that the customer owns and controls their data.

Office 365 follows the regulations protecting the privacy and security of health information, which are enforced by the HIPAA Privacy Rule and the HIPAA Security Rule. The Privacy Rule establishes national standards for the protection of certain health information. The Security Rule establishes a national set of security standards for protecting certain health information that is held or transferred in electronic form. All of Office 365's core services are HIPAA compliant with the signing of a BAA. This BAA includes full Office 365 services—Exchange, SharePoint, Skype for Business, and Office.

HITRUST

The Health Information Trust Alliance (HITRUST) was born out of the belief that information security should be a core pillar of, rather than an obstacle to, the broad adoption of health information systems and exchanges. HITRUST, in collaboration with healthcare, business, technology, and information-security leaders, has established the HITRUST CSF, a certifiable framework that can be used by all organizations that create, access, store, or exchange personal health and financial information.

All the Office 365 core services are compliant with HITRUST, validated by an independent assessor. HITRUST compliance includes full Office 365 services—Exchange, SharePoint, Skype for Business, and Office.

Secure File Sharing

Microsoft Office 365 and OneDrive are compliant and/or certified with the following industry standards/frameworks:

- HITRUST CSF Validated Certification Assessment
- ISO 27001
- ISO 27018
- SSAE16 SOC 1 Type I and Type II and SOC 2 Type II

The HITRUST certification demonstrates that foundational controls are in place to address healthcare-specific regulatory requirements, including HIPAA and HITECH mandates. The HITRUST Common Security Framework is also mapped to the National Institute of Technology (NIST) series of security frameworks, including NIST 800-53 and the NIST Cybersecurity Framework (CSF).

Office 365 provides services near to where you are. It is important to select the correct region for the Office 365 services so that the organization's data doesn't leave the organization's own country. Both HIPAA and HITRUST require healthcare providers to adopt strong password policies, including password length, complexity, and reset settings. It is vital for any healthcare provider to configure Office 365 in this manner so as to follow the regulation standards as well as to follow their own organization's policy standards. Healthcare organizations should also think about configuring multi-factor authentication (MFA) for Office 365 services, as those services will be accessed from outside of the corporate network. MFA will provide an extra layer of security over traditional authentication.

Administrators can use privacy and security options to limit access to files and sensitive information stored in Office 365. Healthcare organizations must develop privacy and security baseline configuration standards to govern the use of data in Office 365. Let's see some examples of the standards providers should set:

- Disable external sharing of sensitive data so that links to the files cannot be sent to email addresses outside of the organization.
- Restrict network access to whitelisted trusted networks only.
- Apply data loss prevention (DLP) rules that prevent files from being accessed by unauthorized users and set up appropriate remediation rules.

- Train users on not sharing files with "everyone" unless necessary. Recommend that files be shared with specific individuals or groups that are authorized to access the files.

- Deactivate users immediately when they leave the organization so that they don't have access to OneDrive and its content.

- Apply conditional access and mobile application management policies to ensure that all devices, regardless of ownership, that connect to OneDrive meet the security and compliance requirements.

- Train users not to store files in OneDrive that contain login and password credentials.

Mobile Device Management

More and more healthcare organizations are adopting mobile usage for their employees as well as developing apps for their patients to provide information quickly. Data collected via mobile apps can be used by providers to get better prepared when there are spikes in outbreaks or disease symptoms.

Organizations can allow information workers or clinicians to access data using their mobile devices from any location. This is particularly helpful for nurses who go to remote locations to provide care and require access to the healthcare information of a patient, including their medical history. Mobile apps such as Epic's Haiku and Canto provide easy access to chart review, patient lists, schedules, and messaging. Nurses can also immediately instant message physicians for consultation and improve patient care during the visit via the Skype for Business app.

Recently, Apple announced the launch of a health records app with HL7's FHIR specifications at 12 hospitals, which will allow patients to view their own medical history, with the hope that this information will help them better understand their health and help them lead healthier lives.[7]

The use of mobile devices also makes it mandatory for healthcare providers to secure data on those mobile devices as per HIPAA regulations. Office 365 supports many Mobile Data Managment (MDM) providers, such as Intune, AirWatch, and MobileIron, that

---

[7]http://www.healthcareitnews.com/news/
apple-launch-health-records-app-hl7s-fhir-specifications-12-hospitals

secure data at rest in mobile devices. MDM uses centralized device security policies to manage and secure the devices automatically. Organizations can use MDM to encrypt the data, force password authentication, and wipe the device remotely if the device is stolen or lost. Organizations can apply conditional access policies to prevent unauthorized access to company network and Petient Health Information (PHI) data; they can also force users to enroll mobile devices into corporate MDM if they want to access sensitive information via Outlook or Office apps (Word, PowerPoint, Excel, Skype, OneNote).

Office 365 MDM security settings include the following:

- Per device application access restriction

- Attachments secured via password

- Apply read, edit, and delete permissions to file

- Require allocation-level passcode for Office 365 apps

- Automatic wipe of device based on number of failed login attempts to prevent brute-force attacks

- Require strong password and expiration policies

- Prevent rooted devices from joining corporate networks

- Apply rights management to prevent screenshots being taken of sensitive information or to block copy/paste from work app to personal app

Data Loss Prevention

Office 365 offers DLP policies to inspect content within a document or email via deep content analysis and block the content if it doesn't match organizational DLP policies.

Office 365 DLP capabilities can be used to do the following:

- Capture sensitive information in email, SharePoint, and OneDrive for Business via regular expression keyword searches

- Prevent users from sharing sensitive information unknowingly

- Provide tooltips and alert messages to users and admins to educate on policy violations and to take appropriate action

- Provide reports to gain visibility into sensitive content stored within SharePoint and OneDrive for Business

Over 55 preconfigured DLP policy templates are available to detect specific types of sensitive information, such as HIPAA data (i.e., PHI), PCI DSS data, or locale-specific personally identifiable information (PII).

Administrators can configure the actions to take based on the conditions met via the DLP engine. DLP can be set on target sites or on specific type of documents. Administrators can configure DLP policy tips to inform email or document senders that they are about to transmit sensitive information that includes PHI. Policy tips can be customized and serve the purpose of educating users and admins on violations of DLP policies and the blocking of messages.

Audit Logging and Monitoring

Office 365 has built-in capabilities for logging and monitoring every activity in all Office 365 services. This supports healthcare organizations' HIPAA compliance obligations for logging and monitoring access to PHI. Audit logging and monitoring helps detect and respond to potential information security-break events by providing an additional security protection layer.

The following types of activities are logged in audit logs that organizations can search easily via the Office 365 Security & Compliance Center or via the PowerShell API:

- User and admin activities in SharePoint Online and OneDrive for Business

- User and admin activities in Exchange Online (Exchange mailbox audit logging)

- Admin activities in Azure Active Directory (the directory service for Office 365)

- User and admin activities in Sway, Planner, Skype for Business, Power BI, Yammer, and Microsoft Teams

Ransomware Attacks

During March 2016, many healthcare providers were infected by the Petya ransomware attack, which encrypts the victim computer's master file table and replaces the master boot record with a ransom note, rendering the computer unusable unless the ransom is paid. By May, it had further evolved to include direct file-encryption capabilities as a failsafe. Ransomware attacks in the healthcare industry are not new; the first ever ransomware attack reported in healthcare was in 1989 by Joseph Popp, PhD, an AIDS researcher, who carried out the attack by distributing 20,000 floppy disks to AIDS researchers spanning more than 90 countries, claiming that the disks contained a program that could analyze an individual's risk of acquiring AIDS using a questionnaire. After 28 years, healthcare providers are still victimized by similar but more sophisticated ransomware attacks.

According to Kaspersky Lab researchers, the top three ransomware families during the first quarter of the year 2016 were Teslacrypt (58.4 percent), CTB-Locker (23.5 percent), and Cryptowall (3.4 percent). All three of these mainly infected users through spam emails with malicious attachments or links to infected web pages. User behavior is the weakest link in exposing organizations to cyberattacks. No matter how much training and education you provide, odds are that there will still be at least one user who will click on the link. Executives often fall into this trap as they do not have time to look beyond the subject of the email, and it requires only one click to spread the virus organization-wide. Most of the ransomware attacks are after valuable patient data. Imagine a doctor comes to the hospital and finds out that his/her work machine is now compromised, due to which all the patient data is now locked up in that workstation, and there is no way to retrieve that data except by paying the ransom. As medical devices are getting more and more connected to the web, and rightfully so, they are getting exposed to cyberthreats more and more. Hackers continue to find creative ways to exploit vulnerabilities, and it can severely cripple hospital operations.

As recently as Friday, May 12, 2017, a new ransomware attack known as WannaCry brought the United Kingdom's National Health Service (NHS) to its knees. In a single day, it was reported to have infected more than 230,000 computers in over 150 countries. WannaCry targeted computers running the Microsoft Windows operating system by encrypting data and demanding ransom payments in the Bitcoin cryptocurrency. This is why health organizations must seriously consider investing in security best practices, and IT should increase its budget to constantly monitor and prevent getting hacked.

Office 365 provides Exchange Advanced Threat Protection (ATP) that can protect healthcare organizations from users who click on random links and get exposed to ransomware attacks. ATP helps by protecting against unsafe attachments and expanding protection against malicious links in order to provide better zero-day protection. ATP helps with safe attachments and safe links so that you can prevent malicious attachments from impacting your messaging environment, even if their signatures are not known. All suspicious content and links go through a real-time behavioral malware analysis that uses machine-learning techniques to evaluate the content for suspicious activity. Unsafe attachments are sandboxed in a detonation chamber before being sent to recipients. The advantage is a malware-free and cleaner inbox with better zero-day attack protection. The URLs are examined in real time as a user clicks them. If a link is unsafe, the user is warned not to visit the site or is informed that the site has been blocked. ATP also provides rich reporting functionality so that admins can analyze and take appropriate action.

Conclusion

Every day, healthcare organizations are faced with increasing pressure to reduce operational costs while still maintaining robust security protections to address emerging threats, regulatory-enforcement activities, and data-breach prevention. Patients are demanding more transparency and better care. Clinicians and nurses want to spend more time with patients by reducing the time they spend on administrative tasks, which they can do by leveraging more automated sophisticated tools. Technological innovations are readily available for any healthcare organization to tap into. All they need to do is reach out and seek those innovations and then provide high-value patient care.

Office 365 has a substantive security portfolio that makes the product a viable option for moving healthcare data to the cloud in a secure and compliant manner. Healthcare organizations will have to get ready for those innovations and must attract a new generation of talent in order to be competitive, much like the financial services industry did. This means that healthcare providers will have to increase the wages and relax the laws to attract younger and brighter talent. It is the time to revolutionize the healthcare industry with better-skilled employees and highly sophisticated tools. In next chapters, we will talk about how you can apply some of your existing investment in Office 365 and maximize the ROI.

CHAPTER 2

Configuring Office 365

Office 365 is a Software as a Service (SaaS) offering from Microsoft. It comes in various licensing models and has specific licenses for small and medium businesses as well as for education-domain customers. This chapter will not focus on the various licensing options of Office 365, but rather will focus on things to remember while configuring Office 365. Office 365 offers a variety of services such as email, shared calendar, document management, team collaboration, mobile access, instant messaging, online meetings, and presence, which are mainly focused around improving the productivity of an organization. We will review some of these services and showcase how to configure them and what to keep in mind when configuring them for a healthcare environment.

Configuration

In this section we will describe the configuration steps for Office 365 for an organization. There are several fundamental architectural pillars that are required, including Azure Active Directory Connect, Active Directory Federation Services, multi-factor authentication, and conditional access. These are described in the "Core Enablement" section. These configurations are a must from the security and governance perspective for any organization. The following sections will also describe how to secure email in Exchange Online and how to configure OneDrive for Business for secure collaboration.

Core Enablement

It is important to make sure that the foundation is built right before we start building the house. Similarly, before you start using Office 365 services, it is important that the foundation at the infrastructure level is rock solid. The following section will discuss the components required and the process to build a strong foundation.

© Nidhish Dhru 2018
N. Dhru, *Office 365 for Healthcare Professionals*, https://doi.org/10.1007/978-1-4842-3549-2_2

Azure Active Directory Connect (AAD Connect)

Office 365 and all its services rely heavily on Azure Active Directory (AAD). AAD is a cloud-based directory and identity-management system. AAD provides an affordable, easy-to-use solution to give employees and business partners single sign-on (SSO) access to thousands of cloud SaaS applications like Office 365. To make single sign-on work, the organization will have to sync its on-premises identities to AAD. A tool that can help with integrating on-premises directories with AAD is AAD Connect. AAD Connect helps users by allowing them to use their on-premises identities to access both on-premises applications and cloud services such as Office 365. There is no need to create a separate identity for Office 365 and no need to worry about managing those identities separately. For more information on the AAD Connect tool, read the article "Integrate Your On-premises Directories with Azure Active Directory."[1]

Before installing or running the AAD Connect tool, an organization will have to make sure that its on-premises Active Directory environment is in a good state for it to be synced with AAD. A tool that can help determine what will break when trying to sync the on-premises directory to AAD is IdFix.

IdFix

IdFix identifies errors such as duplicates and formatting problems in the on-premises Active Directory before synchronizing to AAD. Typically, IdFix throws hundreds of errors if the on-premises Active Directory is not managed properly, and it's advisable to fix those issues before syncing the directory to AAD.

You can learn more about IdFix from the article "Prepare Directory Attributes for Synchronization with Office 365 by Using the IdFix Tool."[2]

---

[1]https://docs.microsoft.com/en-us/azure/active-directory/connect/
active-directory-aadconnect

[2]https://support.office.com/en-us/article/Prepare-directory-attributes-for-synchronization-with-Office-365-by-using-the-IdFix-tool-497593cf-24c6-491c-940b-7c86dcde9de0

Active Directory Federation Services (ADFS)

Another key decision point for any organization is how users will access Office 365. Should the organization allow their users to use a cloud-only identity, meaning they would need a separate Office 365 user ID and password, or use a hybrid identity where the user ID and password for the on-premises Active Directory can be used to access Office 365? In most healthcare organizations, the hybrid identity is the best option considering the ease of use and fewer administration overheads.

Once the identity model is selected, the access model must be chosen. The organization will have to decide how users will use those hybrid identities to log in to Office 365. There are three ways in which users can access Office 365, as follows:

- **Password hash synchronization**: With password hash synchronization, hashes of user passwords are synchronized from on-premises Active Directory to Azure AD. When passwords are changed or reset on-premises, the new password hashes are synchronized to Azure AD immediately so that your users can always use the same password for both cloud resources and on-premises resources. The passwords are never sent to Azure AD or stored in Azure AD in clear text.

- **Pass-through authentication**: With pass-through authentication, the user's password is validated against the on-premises Active Directory controller. The password doesn't need to be present in Azure AD in any form. This allows for on-premises policies, such as sign-in hour restrictions, to be evaluated during authentication to cloud services.

- **Federated Single Sign-On**: With federated sign-on, users can sign in to Azure AD–based services with their on-premises passwords. While users are on the corporate network, they don't even have to enter their passwords.

Most healthcare organizations have security policy constraints that prevent them from storing user passwords anywhere but the on-premises Active Directory, and users don't like the experience of entering their credentials again and again to log in to cloud-based services such as Office 365. That leaves most organizations with one highly secure and most user-friendly choice of federated single sign-on. ADFS helps establish the federated single sign-on between on-premise Active Directory and Azure Active

Directory. By using the federation option, organizations can deploy a new or existing farm with ADFS in Windows Server 2012 R2. Azure AD Connect configures the trust between the ADFS farm and Azure AD so that users can sign in.

Multi-Factor Authentication

Multi-factor authentication (MFA) is a method of authentication that requires the use of more than one verification method and adds a second layer of security to user sign-ins and transactions. It works by requiring any two or more verification methods, such as a randomly generated pass code, a phone call, a smart card (virtual or physical), or a biometric device. When using MFA for Office 365, users are required to acknowledge a phone call, text message, or app notification on their smartphones after correctly entering their passwords. They can sign in only after this second authentication factor has been satisfied. To enable MFA in Office 365, do the following:

1. Sign in to Office 365 with your work account.

2. Go to the Office 365 Admin Center.

3. Navigate to Users ➤ Active users. See Figure 2-1.

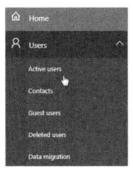

Figure 2-1. *Select "Active users"*

4. In the Office 365 Admin Center, click More ➤ Setup azure multi-factor auth. See Figure 2-2.

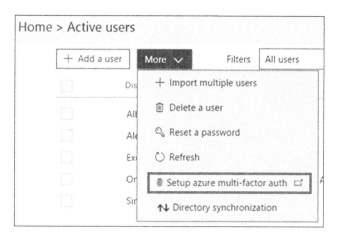

Figure 2-2. *Setup MFA*

5. Find the user or users you want to enable for MFA. In order to see all the users, you might need to change the Multi-Factor Authentication status view at the top.

    The views have the following values based on the MFA state of the users:

    •   Any: Displays all users. This is the default state.

    •   Enabled: The user has been enrolled in multi-factor authentication but has not completed the registration process. They will be prompted to complete the process the next time they sign in.

    •   Enforced: The user may or may not have completed registration. If they have completed the registration process then they are using multi-factor authentication. Otherwise, the user will be prompted to complete the process at next sign-in.

6. Check the checkbox next to the users you want to enable. See Figure 2-3.

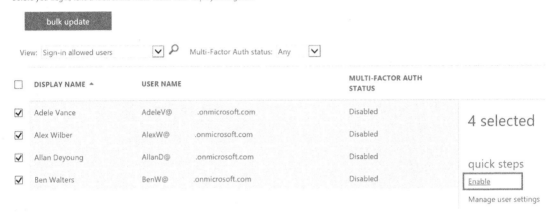

Figure 2-3. Enabling MFA for selected users

7.   On the right user info pane, under quick steps, choose "Enable."

8.   In the dialog box that opens, click "Enable multi-factor auth."

MFA is good for all the browser-based apps, but what happens to apps such as Office 2013, including Outlook? It can be a very annoying experience for users when they try to open either Word or Outlook and apps keep prompting them for MFA or for user name and password, as desktop-based apps use basic authentication. To overcome this challenge, modern authentication has been introduced.

Modern Authentication

Modern authentication brings Active Directory Authentication Library (ADAL)–based sign-in to Office client apps across platforms. This enables sign-in features such as multi-factor authentication (MFA), SAML-based third-party identity providers with Office client applications, and smart card– and certificate-based authentication, and it removes the need for Outlook to use the basic authentication protocol. The Office client will behave exactly as a web browser does when authenticating; it will send the access token requests directly to the authentication provider instead of sending username and password to the resource, and Office client apps will see the exact same behavior with MFA as they do with Office web apps or SharePoint Online. To enable Office 365 modern authentication, see the following for compatibility and default configuration information:

- Modern authentication is automatically on for Office 2016 client apps.

- Office 2013 client apps support legacy authentication by default. *Legacy* means that they support either Microsoft Online Sign-in Assistant or basic authentication. In order for these clients to use modern authentication features, the Windows client has registry keys set. To turn it on for Office 2013 client apps, view the article "Enable Modern Authentication for Office 2013 on Windows Devices."[3]

- For the Office 365 services, the default state of modern authentication is as follows:

  - Exchange Online is on by default.

  - SharePoint Online is on by default.

  - Skype for Business Online is on by default.

Conditional Access

Every organization has policies to prevent users from sharing internal resources externally without protecting them. Conditional access provides the control and protection organizations need to keep corporate data secure while giving employees an experience that allows them to do their best work from any device. More and more organizations are allowing their employees to be productive from anywhere at any time using any device. This also increases the responsibility of the IT and Security department to make sure that the corporate data is highly secure all the time. Conditional access is a capability of Azure Active Directory that enables organizations to enforce controls on access to apps in the corporate environment based on specific conditions. Figure 2-4 shows the conditional access flow.

---

[3]https://support.office.com/en-us/article/Enable-Modern-Authentication-for-Office-2013-on-Windows-devices-7dc1c01a-090f-4971-9677-f1b192d6c910

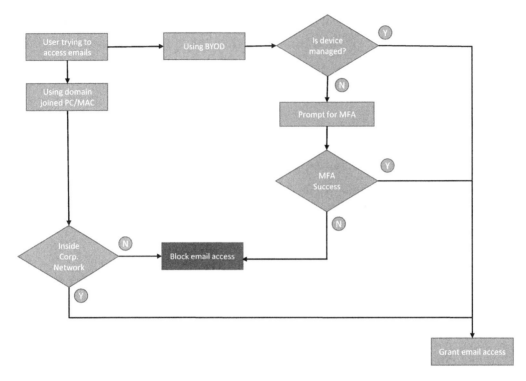

Figure 2-4. *Conditional access flow*

One common requirement in many organizations is to only require multi-factor authentication for access to apps that is not initiated from the corporate intranet. As shown in the preceding diagram, email access should be blocked if the user is trying to access email from their personal PC/MAC from their home. Healthcare organizations might not want their nurses and physicians to access corporate emails from their homes due to regulations. You can address these questions using conditional access. If a nurse is trying to access email from a domain-joined PC from within the hospital, then email should be accessible. If the nurse is trying to access email from a managed device such as a tablet or phone during hospital rounds, then email should be accessible, but if the device is not managed by the organization then prompt for multi-factor authentication before opening the Outlook app. This validates that the right user is accessing the right resources. Follow the steps listed in the article "Get Started with Conditional Access in Azure Active Directory."[4]

---

[4]https://docs.microsoft.com/en-us/azure/active-directory/
active-directory-conditional-access-azure-portal-get-started

Securing Emails

Once the core enablement is completed, it will be the right time to safely migrate on-premises emails from Exchange Server to Office 365 Exchange Online. The migration process will be different based on the existing version of on-premises Exchange Server. For migrations from an existing on-premises Exchange Server environment, an administrator can migrate all email, calendar, and contacts from user mailboxes to Office 365. There are several approaches to migrating mailboxes to Exchange Online. View the article "Ways to Migrate Multiple Email Accounts to Office 365" for all the techniques of email migration.[5]

Exchange Online Protection (EOP)

Microsoft Exchange Online Protection (EOP) is a cloud-based email-filtering service that helps protect organizations against spam and malware and includes features to safeguard organizations from messaging-policy violations. Once emails are moved to Exchange Online, it is important to protect incoming emails from malware. See Figure 2-5 for the EOP process flow.

---

[5]https://support.office.com/en-us/article/Ways-to-migrate-multiple-email-accounts-to-Office-365-0a4913fe-60fb-498f-9155-a86516418842

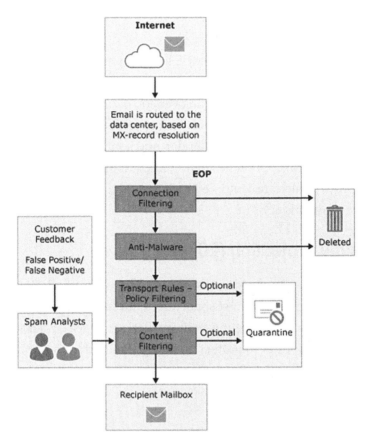

Figure 2-5. *EOP process flow[6]*

After EOP is configured, an incoming message initially passes through connection filtering, which checks the sender's reputation and inspects the message for malware. Most spam is stopped at this point and deleted by EOP. Messages continue through policy filtering, where they are evaluated against custom transport rules that you create or enforce from a template. For example, you can have a rule that sends a notification to a manager when mail arrives from a specific sender. Next, messages pass through content filtering, where content is checked for terminology or properties common to spam. A message determined to be spam by the content filter can be sent to a user's Junk Email folder or to quarantine, among other options, based on your settings. After a message passes these protection layers successfully, it is delivered to the recipient. View the article "Exchange Online Protection Overview" to learn more about how to configure EOP.[7]

---

[6]https://technet.microsoft.com/en-us/library/jj723119(v=exchg.150).aspx
[7]https://technet.microsoft.com/en-us/library/jj723119(v=exchg.150).aspx

Advanced Threat Protection (ATP)

ATP is an email-filtering technology that prevents zero-day cyberattacks by providing additional protection against unknown malware/ransomware and viruses; real-time, time-of-click protection against malicious URLs and phishing attacks; and rich reporting and URL trace capabilities. Office 365 offers this robust protection for customers as an optional add-on to their existing service or as part of the new E5 suite to protect organizations against increasingly sophisticated attacks. ATP safe links can help protect your organization according to policies that are set by your Office 365 security administrators. Policies are set for specific people or groups, or for the entire organization. ATP safe links protection can apply to hyperlinks in emails and hyperlinks in Office documents, such as Word, Excel, PowerPoint, and Visio files on Windows. View the article "Set Up Office 365 ATP Safe Links Policies" to learn how to set up safe links.[8]

DLP

To comply with business standards and industry regulations, healthcare organizations need to protect sensitive information and prevent its inadvertent disclosure. Examples of sensitive information that organizations might want to prevent from leaking outside the organization include financial data or personally identifiable information (PII) such as credit card numbers, social security numbers, medical record numbers (MRN), or health records. With a data loss prevention (DLP) policy in the Office 365 Security & Compliance Center, an organization can identify, monitor, and automatically protect sensitive information across Office 365. Data loss prevention (DLP) is a strategy for making sure that employees at a healthcare organization do not share sensitive or critical information outside the corporate network.

DLP policies can help

- identify sensitive information across many locations, such as Exchange Online, SharePoint Online, and OneDrive for Business;

- prevent the accidental sharing of sensitive information;

- monitor and protect sensitive information in the desktop versions of Excel 2016, PowerPoint 2016, and Word 2016;

---

[8]https://support.office.com/en-us/article/Set-up-ATP-safe-links-policies-in-Office-365-bdd5372d-775e-4442-9c1b-609627b94b5d

- teach users how to stay compliant without interrupting their workflow; and

- view DLP reports showing content that matches your organization's DLP policies.

For creating and managing DLP policies, go to the data loss prevention page in the Office 365 Security & Compliance Center as shown in Figure 2-6.

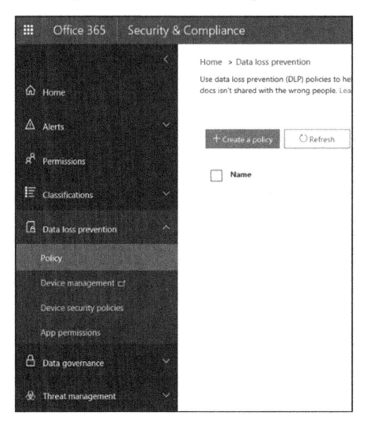

Figure 2-6. *Create new DLP policy*

Exchange Online DLP policies can be set up to notify users that they are sending sensitive information or to block the transmission of sensitive information. Exchange Online has flexible and customizable rule configurations, exclusions (e.g., Document Fingerprint), and end-user notifications. Office 365 also has full DLP features implemented for OneDrive for Business and SharePoint Online, including the ability to define/apply policies, detect external sharing and take action, detect based on metadata, notify users with policy tips or email, and so on. Office 365 DLP policies are also synched to the local machine with Office 2016.

Configure SharePoint Online

SharePoint Online is a cloud-based service that helps organizations share and collaborate with colleagues, partners, and customers. With SharePoint Online, users can access internal sites, documents, and other information from anywhere—at the office, at home, or from a mobile device. SharePoint Online does not require any on-premises infrastructure except the components previously mentioned in the "Core Enablement" section. An Office 365 global administrator can go to the SharePoint Online portal using their work account and create sites on which users can start collaborating. The Office 365 global administrator must assign SharePoint Online licenses first before users can start interacting with the newly created SharePoint sites. To assign SharePoint Online licenses to users, do the following:

1. Sign in to Office 365 (`https://portal.office.com/`) using the global administrator account.

2. Go to Admin Center and click on "Active users"; see Figure 2-7.

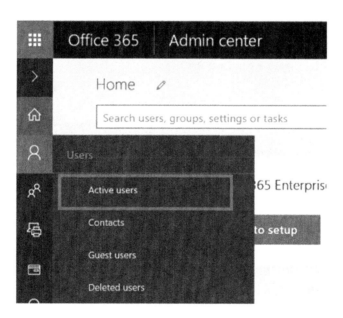

Figure 2-7. *Go to list of active users*

3. Select a user or users for which a license needs to be assigned and click on "Edit licenses" as shown in Figure 2-8.

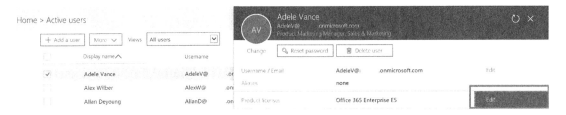

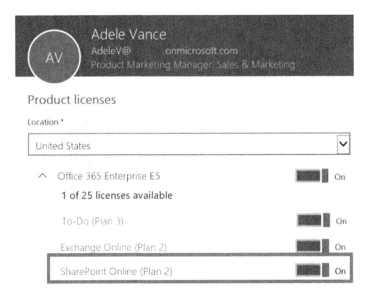

Figure 2-8. *Edit user product licenses*

4. Turn on the SharePoint Online license for that user and click
    "Save" as shown in Figure 2-9.

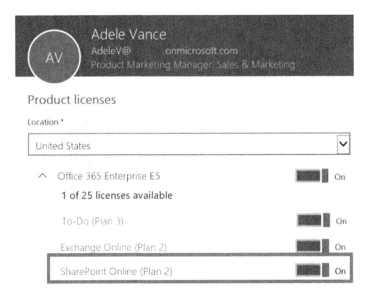

Figure 2-9. *Assigning SharePoint license to user*

Once the license is assigned and the administrator gives the user access to a
SharePoint Online site, users can start collaborating on that site. These steps can also
be automated for the entire organization using a PowerShell script, as described in the
article "Assign Licenses to User Accounts with Office 365 PowerShell."[9]

---

[9]https://technet.microsoft.com/en-us/library/dn771770.aspx

A SharePoint Online global administrator can create team sites using the SharePoint Online Admin Portal and assign permissions to administer the site. To create a team site, a SharePoint administrator can do the following:

1. Go to `https://{your domain}-admin.sharepoint.com`

2. Click on New ➤ Private Site Collection as shown in Figure 2-10.

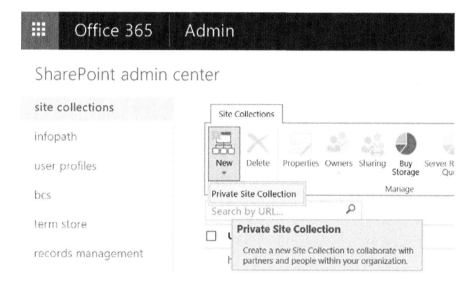

Figure 2-10. *Create private site collection*

3. Enter all the relevant information and click "Save." A new site will be created in a few minutes as shown in Figure 2-11.

41

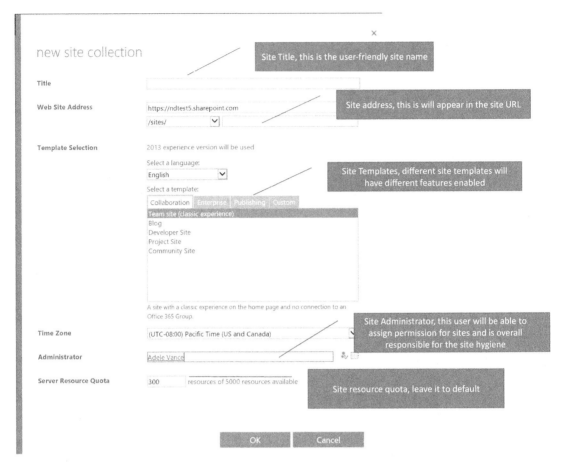

Figure 2-11. *Site collection attributes*

In few minutes, the site will be ready for use. The administrator can also create sites using PowerShell.

Configure OneDrive for Business

OneDrive for Business is the personal storage location for enterprise users. The contents of this library can optionally be synchronized with one or more of the user's computers or devices. By using OneDrive for Business, organizations can ensure that business files for their users are stored in a central location, which makes it easy for users to share and collaborate on documents. Office 365 can also reduce the on-premises storage costs by moving users' files to the cloud. For enterprise users, Office 365 offers unlimited storage for more than five users. Initially, storage is capped at 5 TB per user, but organizations can request additional storage for users if needed. OneDrive for Business is a personalized site from SharePoint Online, so once you have configured SharePoint Online, OneDrive for Business is configured as an SaaS service. After that, users have two choices to store and access files:

1. Access OneDrive for Business from browser:

    a. Click on OneDrive from the waffle menu at the top-left corner of the Office 365 portal as shown in Figure 2-12.

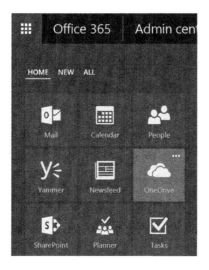

Figure 2-12. *Go to OneDrive for Business Portal*

    b. User will be redirected to `https://***-my.sharepoint.com/ personal/{user}_***_onmicrosoft_com/_layouts/15/ onedrive.aspx` as shown in Figure 2-13.

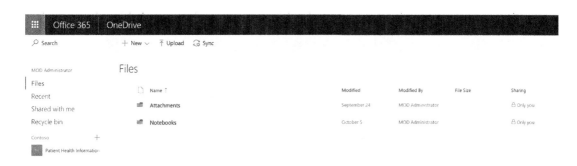

Figure 2-13. *User's OneDrive for Business portal*

From here, users can start uploading and viewing documents as their personal storage for official use.

2. Access OneDrive for Business from a sync client:

   a. Install the OneDrive for Business client from `https://oneclient.sfx.ms/Win/Direct/17.3.6281.1202/OneDriveSetup.exe` as shown in Figure 2-14.

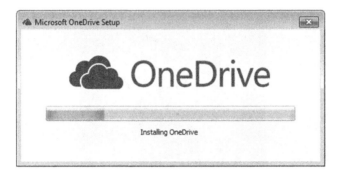

Figure 2-14. *Downloading OneDrive for Business*

   b. Once the client is installed, sign in to Office 365 and chose which folders to sync to OneDrive for Business, as shown in Figure 2-15.

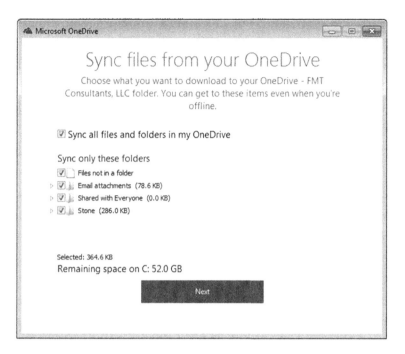

Figure 2-15. *Syncing folders to OneDrive for Business*

Once the folders are synced, the sync client will automatically sync all the changes back up to Office 365.

Securing Documents

Office 365 provides a platform for security and compliance across all its services, such as SharePoint Online, OneDrive for Business, and Exchange Online. The configured DLP policies for Exchange Online will also work for SharePoint Online and OneDrive for Business. Office 365 also offers labeling and information protection with Information Rights Management (IRM). IRM protects sensitive information from unauthorized access via Exchange Online and SharePoint/OneDrive for Business. Exchange Online IRM controls such actions as forwarding, extracting information, saving files, or sending an email. SharePoint and OneDrive for Business are IRM-enabled at a file level, regardless of where it is later stored, which means only authorized people can view them. Common restrictions that can be applied to these files include making them read-only, disabling the copying of text, preventing people from saving a local copy, and preventing people from printing the file. Information protection via labeling is a new concept in Office documents. Each label is tied to the IRM policy, which makes it easier for users to identify the correct label for a document from the get-go. Chapter 7, "Personal Health Record External Sharing Securely," will describe how to prevent users from sharing sensitive information externally by using DLP, IRM, and information Protection in Office 365.

OneDrive for Business and SharePoint Online both protect documents both at rest and in transit. Communication with OneDrive for Business across the internet uses SSL/TLS connections. All SSL connections are established using 2048-bit keys. Encryption at rest includes two components: BitLocker disk-level encryption and per-file encryption of customer content. While BitLocker encrypts all data on a disk, per-file encryption goes even further by including a unique encryption key for each file. Every update to every file is encrypted using its own encryption key. Before they're stored, the keys to the encrypted content are stored in a physically separate location from the content. Every step of this encryption uses Advanced Encryption Standard (AES) with 256-bit keys and is Federal Information Processing Standard (FIPS) 140-2 compliant. The encrypted content is distributed across many containers throughout the data center, and each container has unique credentials. These credentials are stored in a separate physical location from both the content and the content keys.

Working Offline on Documents

OneDrive for Business allows you to create or edit a document from a mobile device or personal computer that is not connected to the internet. Office 365 offers offline editing capabilities from its rich client apps, which helps ensure version control is no longer a concern. Resolving conflicting changes is a feature enabled on files stored, shared, and worked on from OneDrive for Business (online or offline). This capability helps users know exactly what final version is being saved for future use. This feature is useful when nurses or physicians have synced the documents into their local devices and must access them even if the internet is not available. The OneDrive for Business sync client makes sure that offline and online versions are always in sync. Once the documents are modified offline, the sync client will update the changes in the background once the internet connection is available.

Configuring Microsoft TEAMS

Microsoft TEAMS is a new chat-based workspace in Office 365. It is an entirely new experience that brings together people, conversations, and content, along with the tools that teams need, so they can easily collaborate to achieve more. Chapter 5, "Innovations in Tumor Board Reviews," talks about all the features and functionality of MS TEAMS and how to best use it in a clinical environment. The following section will show you how to configure MS TEAMS in Office 365 tenant:

1. Sign in to Office 365 with your administrator account.

2. Select "Admin" to go to the Office 365 Admin Center.

3. From Settings, select "Services & add-ins" or "Apps" as shown in Figure 2-16.

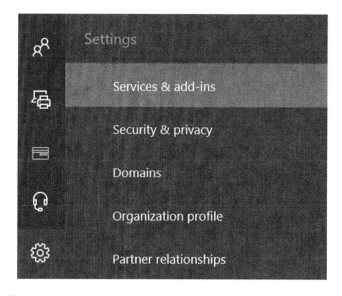

Figure 2-16. *Office 365 Services & Add-ins page*

4. From the list of services and add-ins, or apps, select "Microsoft Teams" as shown in Figure 2-17.

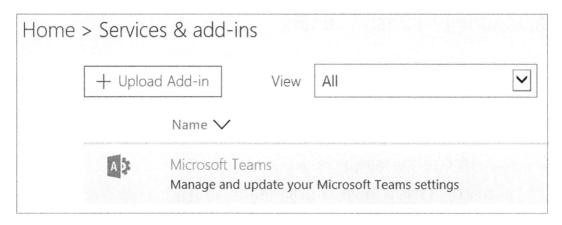

Figure 2-17. *Update Teams settings*

5. On the Microsoft Teams settings screen, switch Microsoft Teams to *On* and then select "Save" as shown in Figure 2-18.

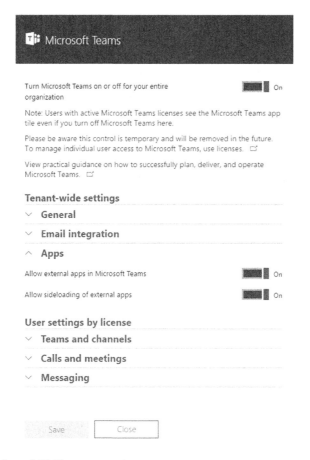

Figure 2-18. *Update MS Teams settings*

Once the configuration is done, users can start using MS Teams as shown in Figure 2-19.

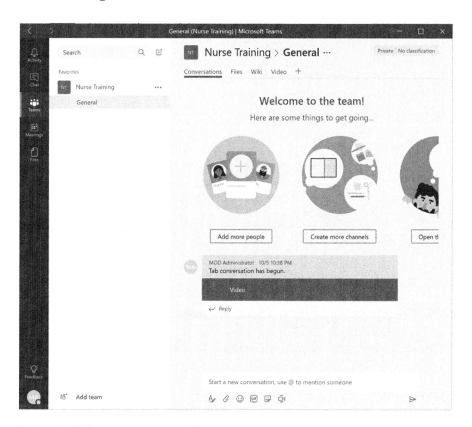

Figure 2-19. *MS Teams user interface*

Configuring Skype for Business

Skype for Business is the Office 365 service that allows users to instant message as well as to make voice or video calls. For configuring presence and instant messaging with internal or external users, follow these steps:

1. Sign in to Office 365 with your administrator account.

2. Select "Admin" to go to the Office 365 Admin Center.

3. Click on "Skype for Business" from Admin Center.

4. Click on "Organization," then click on "Automatically display presence information," as shown in Figure 2-20.

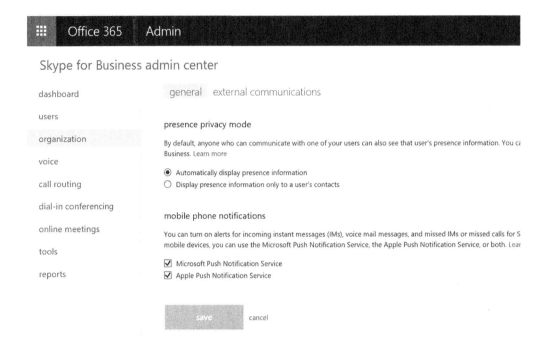

Figure 2-20. *Configure Skype for Business settings*

This should enable the presence status—for example, Available, Away, Do Not Disturb, or Offline—to let others know the user's availability.

5. Click on "External Communication" if you want to allow collaboration with external users, as shown in Figure 2-21.

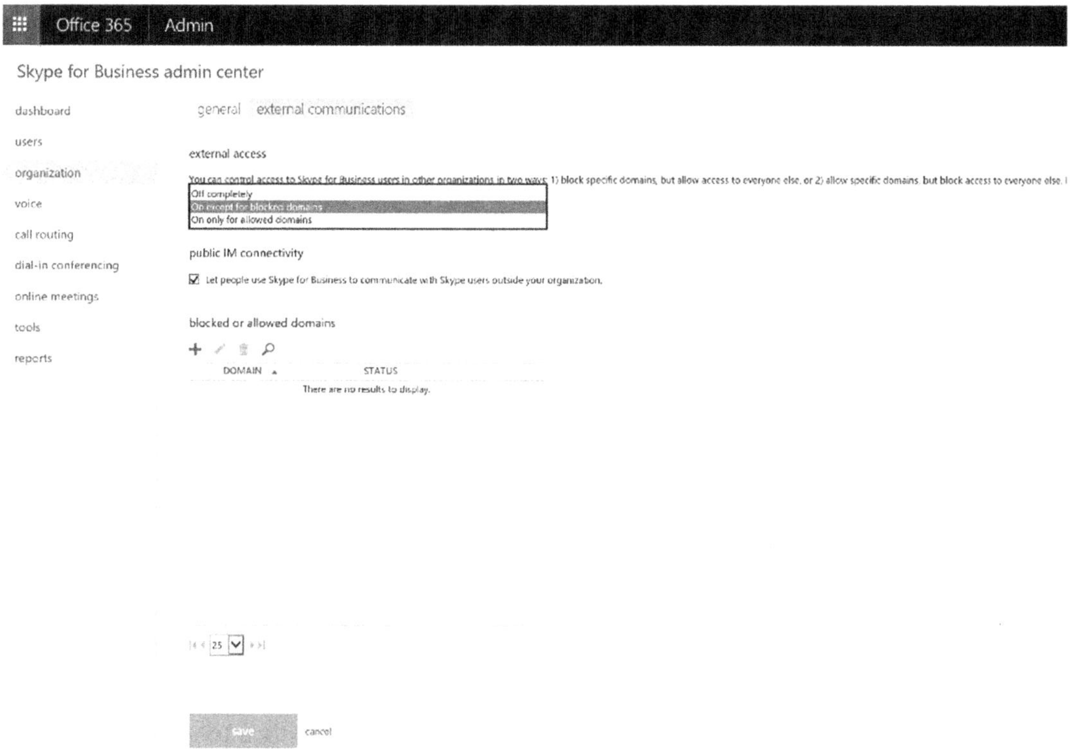

Figure 2-21. *Configure external communication for Skype for Business*

Select options appropriately for your organization. Read the article "Set Up Skype for Business Online" for more information on how to configure each of the Skype for Business Online features.[10]

---

[10]https://support.office.com/en-us/article/
Set-up-Skype-for-Business-Online-40296968-e779-4259-980b-c2de1c044c6e

51

Conclusion

As discussed in this chapter, there are many services in Office 365, and each month new services are being added. Office 365 is an SaaS-based service, which means that with a couple clicks your organization can start using those services. Recently, there were new services added like PowerApps and Flow.

PowerApps allows you to create mobile apps that run on Android, iOS, Windows (Modern Apps), and through almost any internet browser. PowerApps provides a nice drag-and-drop GUI to allow you to add different controls (i.e., text field, choice field, and so forth), media (images, video, camera controls for your phone), forms, and screens to construct a mobile app. It also allows you to connect to external data sources or store data directly inside the app. Once the app is created, users can publish it so it is made available to Android, iOS, and Windows operating systems, as PowerApps takes care of rendering the application no matter what device and browser users are trying to view it on. PowerApps helps you save on development work, support costs, and development resources you need to create business apps.

Similarly, Flow helps you set up automated workflows between your favorite apps and services to synchronize files, get notifications, collect data, and more. With PowerApps and Microsoft Flow, you can connect to data sources like Office 365, SharePoint, Dropbox, Twitter, and other common SaaS and enterprise services. Office 365 continuously makes these investments to keep users very productive using any device at any place.

Overall, Office 365 aims to offer a powerful and flexible set of cloud application services that include a broad range of security features. As more security features are added, with additional configuration capabilities offered for consumers, organizations that transition to Office 365 in the coming years will find that its security is more than capable of meeting most enterprises' needs. In next chapter, we will discuss how organizations can stay compliant while using Office 365 services, remaining productive while being highly secure.

CHAPTER 3

Innovate While Staying Compliant

We live in a highly connected and complex world today. Digital technology as a change agent has enabled us to innovate faster and more cost-effectively to accomplish new goals and achieve new efficiencies. Innovations are no longer region- or country-centric; they are based on data and information from across the world. Innovation is dependent on data, and maintaining and managing that data securely is the responsibility of every citizen and organization. Connected devices and services have provided organizations with valuable data, creating new opportunities to personalize service and drive new business models. This growth is being driven by an ever-increasing number of sources, and the data being generated now is more complex than ever. In many cases, this data-collection process evolved over years across multiple IT systems with variable levels of security and compliance. The amount of electronic data being created by organizations is growing exponentially.

With this new technology comes new challenges and public debates. As business grows, staying compliant in a sea of new global regulations adds new layers of complexity. This has made data governance, regulatory compliance, and eDiscovery some of the most essential business priorities in IT. The rules and regulations that we use to govern technology are also evolving, creating complicated requirements with sometimes blurry boundaries and outcomes. This has simultaneously raised new security and privacy concerns, which the General Data Protection Regulation (GDPR) is responding to. It doesn't matter whether data is created, processed, stored, managed, and protected on desktops, mobile devices, on-premises servers, or in the cloud; the compliance standards essentially hold your organization to the same standard across all your IT environments. Often, these point solutions don't share any information as they are not integrated, which leads to the most dangerous of these challenges: ineffective responses to threats that grow both in number and sophistication and target your organization and

© Nidhish Dhru 2018
N. Dhru, *Office 365 for Healthcare Professionals*, https://doi.org/10.1007/978-1-4842-3549-2_3

your customers. Having more solutions to deploy and more vendors to manage, with less insight and ineffective threat response, ultimately manifests itself in higher costs of security for Chief Information Security Officer (CISOs) as well. An effective security-management solution is not about a single console. Effective security management integrates where it counts and also offers specialized tools for different functions.

Many organizations are exposing themselves to unnecessary risk because they don't have a good grasp on all the data they have. For example, many organizations continue to retain the personal information of former employees who left the company long ago. Were this data to be compromised in a breach, the company could be liable for costly remediation, such as lifetime credit monitoring, for these former employees. While following compliance, legal, and overall governance requirements, organizations must still get business done. Ensuring that users can quickly access the appropriate information when and how they need it is paramount to staying in business. The ability to find information quickly, share knowledge, and make informed decisions can determine an organization's ability to remain agile. Finally, it is essential to consider how you protect content from global cyber threats and the very visible impact of leaks and breaches.

GDPR is one of many regulations and industry standards that an organization may be required to meet and is why Microsoft has been investing more in security and compliance. There are ISO standards for information security management (ISO/IEC 27001) and for cloud privacy (ISO/IEC 27018). Microsoft has implemented a security standard designed to prevent fraud through increased control of credit card data (PCI DSS) and supported a US healthcare law that establishes requirements for the use, disclosure, and safeguarding of individually identifiable health information (HIPAA). Office 365 offers a unique approach with in-place solutions that don't require additional steps or risks to meet the various requirements of different teams. With advanced processing capabilities, tools can draw correlations and take action within the data in a way that an individual would not be able to. The Office 365 Security & Compliance Center has brought these together in a single place to help organizations meet data-governance needs.

Health Insurance Portability and Accountability Act (HIPAA)

In 1996, the Health Insurance Portability and Accountability Act (HIPAA) was endorsed by the US Congress. The HIPAA Privacy Rule, also called the Standards for Privacy of Individually Identifiable Health Information, provided the first nationally recognized regulations for the use/disclosure of an individual's health information. Essentially, the Privacy Rule defines how covered entities (health plan, healthcare clearinghouse, healthcare provider) use individually identifiable health information or PHI (personal health information). HIPAA gives patients control over the use of their health information, defines boundaries for the use/disclosure of health records by covered entities, establishes national standards that healthcare providers must comply with, helps to limit the use of PHI and minimizes chances of its inappropriate disclosure, strictly investigates compliance-related issues and holds violators accountable with civil or criminal penalties for violating the privacy of an individual's PHI, and supports the cause of not disclosing PHI without individual consent for individual healthcare needs, public benefit, and national interests. HIPAA also provides the ability to transfer and continue health insurance coverage for millions of American workers and their families when they change or lose their jobs, and it reduces healthcare fraud and abuse. The HIPAA Privacy regulations require healthcare providers and organizations, as well as their business associates, to develop and follow procedures that ensure the confidentiality and security of protected health information (PHI) when it is transferred, received, handled, or shared. This applies to all forms of PHI, including paper, oral, and electronic. Furthermore, only the minimum health information necessary to conduct business is to be used or shared.

Business Associate Agreement (BAA)

Under the US Health Insurance Portability and Accountability Act of 1996, a HIPAA business associate agreement (BAA) is a contract between a HIPAA-covered entity and a HIPAA business associate (BA). The contract protects personal health information (PHI) in accordance with HIPAA guidelines. According to the Department of Health and Human Services (HHS), examples of HIPAA business associates include the use of third-party administrators to help with claims processing; CPA firms providing account services to healthcare providers and having access to protected health information; consultants performing utilization reviews; healthcare clearinghouses translating claims from a nonstandard format to a standard format for a healthcare provider then sending the processed transaction to a payer; independent medical transcription services; and pharmacy benefits managers who manage a health plan's pharmacist network.

ISO 27001 Certification

ISO 27001 is the best-known international information security standard. Certification provides independent assurance that a provider's staff can effectively operate a comprehensive security program and manage information-security risks effectively. The audit process involves detailed interviews and examination of topics such as physical security, access control, risk management, business continuity, and security best practices during software development. The thorough audit should conclude that the provider's information security management system (ISMS) meets the rigorous physical, logical, process, and management controls required to achieve compliance with the standard.

Office 365 Compliance with HIPAA and BAA

Many of the Microsoft Office 365 offerings are certified under ISO 27001 by independent auditors. The scope of the ISO 27001 audits includes HIPAA security practices as recommended by the US Department of Health and Human Services. Prior to placing ePHI in the online service, organizations should read the HIPAA and BAA documents from Office 365 in full and evaluate themselves as to whether the BAA meets their needs and whether they should place ePHI in Microsoft Office 365. Again, it is ultimately the organization's responsibility to evaluate whether the Office 365 services match their HIPAA implementation strategy requirements and to ensure their personnel use these services in a way that complies with HIPAA requirements. To help comply with HIPAA and the HITECH Act, customers may enter into written agreements with Microsoft called business associate agreements, or BAAs. Microsoft does not require customers to sign BAAs. Instead, Microsoft makes a HIPAA BAA available automatically to all customers with an online service contract in the Online Services Terms. The BAA includes the full spectrum of Office 365 services—Exchange, SharePoint, Skype for Business, Office, and Yammer. Office 365 also provides many security tools to make sure the data inside Office 365 is secure and meets all compliance standards.

- **Encryption at rest and in transit**: Microsoft applies encryption-in-transit to the transfer of information outside of Microsoft facilities. Encryption-in-transit only applies to information that can be encrypted without interfering with standard internet protocols. This means packet headers and message headers are not encrypted in transit, since that would interfere with the delivery of the information. It is strongly recommended that organizations train and instruct their personnel to follow industry-standard HIPAA security guidance to never put ePHI in the "from," "to," or "subject line" fields of an email message.

- **Multi-factor authentication (MFA)**: Office 365 offers multi-factor authentication if organizations choose to implement it. The administrator can configure Office 365 to receive MFA via text, phone call, certificate, or special code. The administrator can configure the policy to prompt for MFA when the user is coming from a non-trusted network or device; otherwise, it will use single sign-on to let users authenticate using their NT LAN Manager (NTLM) credentials. MFA can also be integrated with on-premises third-party MFA providers to hard token support or for any other special requirements.

- **Security breaches**: Upon becoming aware of a security breach involving ePHI, Microsoft will report this to all global administrators on the accounts, to all global or technical administrators, or to the individual administrator acting as the HIPAA administrative contact. In addition, because Microsoft does not scan or otherwise interpret customers' data stored in the services, Microsoft will likely be aware only that a repository appropriate for storage of ePHI has been compromised. The customer will need to determine whether ePHI was present in the dataset subject to the security breach. Microsoft will report information it has developed on any ePHI involved in a security breach within 30 days of the breach. Microsoft relies on the customer to handle all notifications to affected individuals.

- **Exchange Online**: Exchange Online Protection (EOP) will help you configure out-of-the-box rules to enable your clients to be HIPAA compliant. This is done using data loss prevention (DLP) policies. Microsoft Exchange Online Protection (EOP) is a cloud-based email-filtering service that helps protect organizations against spam and malware and includes features to safeguard the organization from messaging-policy violations. EOP can simplify the management of the messaging environment and alleviate many of the burdens that come with maintaining on-premises hardware and software.

DLP policies are simple rules that contain sets of conditions that are made up of transport rules, actions, and exceptions that is created in the Exchange Administration Portal and then activated to filter email messages. Chapter 2 describes how to configure EOP and DLP in detail.

- **SharePoint Online and OneDrive for Business**: Data-leak prevention (DLP) policies and Azure Information Protection (AIP) help with the protecting, monitoring, and blocking of documents for unauthorized access. AIP powered by a rights management service (RMS) can make sure that only those who have permission to view or edit the documents have access to those documents. The eDiscovery feature helps discover documents that don't meet compliance standards and puts them on hold. A hold on a document is transparent from the users, who can view/edit the document without noticing that their document is put on hold. Chapter 7 has detailed information on how to securely collaborate using SharePoint Online.

- **Skype for Business Online**: Skype for Business (SFB) Online allows users to communicate within or outside of their organization via chat or audio or video calls. SFB also allows users to share files and screens with other users. SFB can store all the conversations between users as well as meetings. Per compliance policy, if an organization wants to block these features from SFB Online then the administrator must either use PowerShell or go to the SFB Online admin portal (Figure 3-1).

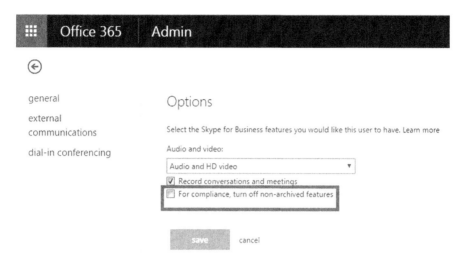

Figure 3-1. Skype for Business Online administration portal

- The preceding setting will turn off features like file transfer using instant messaging, shared OneNote pages, and PowerPoint annotations. The administrator can also block external communications to minimize the PHI data leakage from the same SFB admin center (Figure 3-2).

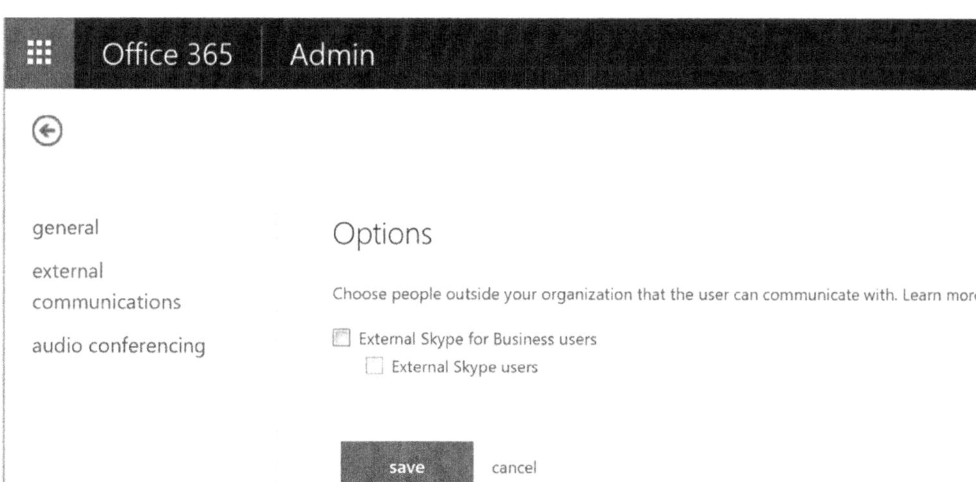

Figure 3-2. Skype for Business Online, turn off external communication

- **Yammer**: Yammer received ISO/IEC 27001:2005 certification by the British Standards Institution (BSI), the national standards body of the United Kingdom, and one of the premier accreditation firms in the world. An organization can acquire a Yammer Data Processing Agreement (DPA) from Microsoft; the DPA addresses the privacy, security, and handling of customer data. Yammer supports SAML 1.1/2.0–based SSO on all web, desktop, and mobile clients. All connections to Yammer are secured via SSL/TLS. Any attempt to connect over HTTP is redirected to HTTPS. Yammer is operated out of Microsoft's global network of datacenters, which have 24/7/365 video surveillance, biometric and pin-based locks, strict personnel access controls, and detailed visitor entry logs. Yammer classifies and treats all data as confidential, using inbound and outbound low-level logical firewalls to ensure that data cannot be leaked between Yammer networks. Sensitive production data is never migrated or used outside of the production network. Yammer has functionality like Skype for Business Online, where external users can join the Yammer network for collaboration. For compliance and privacy restrictions, organizations can block users from creating external Yammer groups so that no data is shared with external users (Figure 3-3).

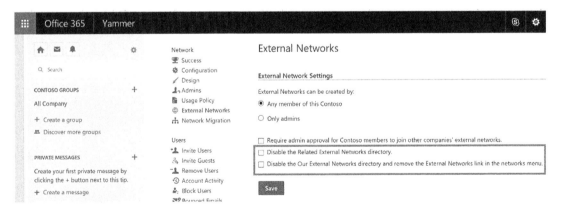

Figure 3-3. *Yammer administration screen, disable external groups*

- **MS Teams**: MS Teams was Tier C–compliant at launch and is compliant with standards such as ISO 27001, ISO 27018, SSAE16 SOC 1 and SOC 2, HIPAA, and EU Model Clauses (EUMC). MS Teams enforces team-wide and organization-wide two-factor authentication, single sign-on through Active Directory, and encryption of data both in transit and at rest. Files are stored in SharePoint and are backed by SharePoint encryption. Notes are stored in OneNote and are backed by OneNote encryption. MS Teams supports the auditing and reporting of audit logs right into the Office 365 Security & Compliance Center. Content Search can be used to search Microsoft Teams through rich filtering capabilities and results can be exported to a specific container for compliance and litigation support. This can be done with or without an eDiscovery case. MS Team capabilities include case management and the preservation, search, analysis, and export of Teams data, including chat, messaging, and file data. When any Team within Microsoft Teams is put on In-Place Hold or Litigation Hold, the hold is placed on the group's mailbox.

Health Information Trust Alliance (HITRUST)

The Health Information Trust Alliance (HITRUST) was born out of the belief that information security should be a core pillar of, rather than an obstacle to, the broad adoption of health information systems and exchanges. HITRUST, in collaboration with healthcare, business, technology, and information-security leaders, created and maintains the Common Security Framework (CSF), a certifiable framework that helps healthcare organizations and their providers demonstrate their security and compliance in a consistent and streamlined manner. CSF can be used by all organizations that create, access, store, or exchange personal health and financial information. The CSF builds on HIPAA and the HITECH Act, which are US healthcare laws that have established requirements for the use, disclosure, and safeguarding of individually identifiable health information and that enforce compliance. HITRUST provides a benchmark—a standardized compliance framework, assessment, and certification process—against which cloud-service providers and covered health entities can measure compliance. The CSF also incorporates healthcare-specific security, privacy, and other regulatory requirements from such existing frameworks as the Payment Card Industry Data Security Standard (PCI-DSS), ISO/IEC 27001 information security management standards, and Minimum Acceptable Risk Standards for Exchanges (MARS-E).

All the Office 365 core services are compliant with HITRUST, which is validated by an independent assessor. HITRUST compliance includes the full spectrum of Office 365 services—Exchange, SharePoint, Skype for Business, Office, and Yammer.

General Data Protection Regulation (GDPR)

The GDPR imposes rules on organizations that offer goods and services to people in the European Union (EU) or that collect and analyze data tied to EU residents, no matter where they are located. These regulations include enhanced personal privacy rights with more flexible controls for individuals to access and interact with their personal data; increased duty for protecting data, including stricter guidelines for confidentiality and recordkeeping and more transparent policies for data handling, mandatory breach reporting, privacy personnel training, and the appointment of a data protection officer (in larger organizations); and significant penalties for non-compliance, including substantial fines that apply whether an organization has intentionally or inadvertently failed to comply. Companies of all sizes and industries need to protect their sensitive data and ensure that it doesn't get into the wrong hands. Employees are using more SaaS apps, creating more data, and working across multiple devices. While this has enabled people to do more, it has also increased the risk of data loss; it is estimated that 58 percent of workers have accidentally shared sensitive data with the wrong person.

The GDPR considers personal data to be any information related to an identified or identifiable natural person. That can include both direct identification (e.g., your legal name) and indirect identification (i.e., specific information that makes it clear it is you the data references, such as SSN). The GDPR makes it clear that the concept of personal data includes online identifiers (e.g., IP addresses, mobile device IDs) and location data, where the EU Data Protection Directive had previously been somewhat unclear. The GDPR introduces specific definitions for genetic data (e.g., an individual's gene sequence) and biometric data. Genetic and biometric data along with other sub-categories of personal data (personal data revealing racial or ethnic origin, political opinions, religious or philosophical beliefs, or trade union membership; data concerning health; or data concerning a person's sex life or sexual orientation) are treated as sensitive personal data under the GDPR. Sensitive personal data is afforded enhanced protections and generally requires an individual's explicit consent where these data are to be processed. Ultimately, your compliance with the GDPR will be determined by how effective your data-governance program is. Organizations need to protect their content and be prepared for internal audits, external litigation, regulatory data requests, and eDiscovery. Human beings, using manual processes, just cannot keep up with this given the likely explosion of personal data across the organization.

Microsoft designed Office and Office 365 with industry-leading security measures and privacy policies to safeguard organizations' data in the cloud, including the categories of personal data identified by the GDPR. Office and Office 365 can help organizations in their journey to reducing risks and achieving compliance with the GDPR (Figure 3-4).

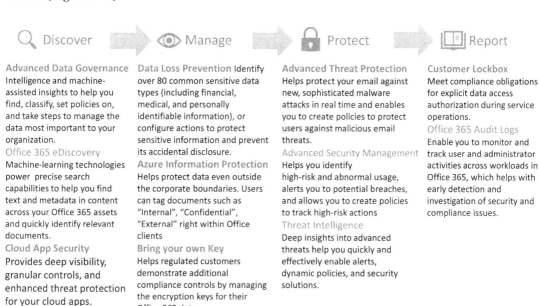

Discover

Advanced Data Governance Intelligence and machine-assisted insights to help you find, classify, set policies on, and take steps to manage the data most important to your organization.

Office 365 eDiscovery Machine-learning technologies power precise search capabilities to help you find text and metadata in content across your Office 365 assets and quickly identify relevant documents.

Cloud App Security Provides deep visibility, granular controls, and enhanced threat protection for your cloud apps.

Manage

Data Loss Prevention Identify over 80 common sensitive data types (including financial, medical, and personally identifiable information), or configure actions to protect sensitive information and prevent its accidental disclosure.

Azure Information Protection Helps protect data even outside the corporate boundaries. Users can tag documents such as "Internal", "Confidential", "External" right within Office clients

Bring your own Key Helps regulated customers demonstrate additional compliance controls by managing the encryption keys for their Office 365 data.

Protect

Advanced Threat Protection Helps protect your email against new, sophisticated malware attacks in real time and enables you to create policies to protect users against malicious email threats.

Advanced Security Management Helps you identify high-risk and abnormal usage, alerts you to potential breaches, and allows you to create policies to track high-risk actions

Threat Intelligence Deep insights into advanced threats help you quickly and effectively enable alerts, dynamic policies, and security solutions.

Report

Customer Lockbox Meet compliance obligations for explicit data access authorization during service operations.

Office 365 Audit Logs Enable you to monitor and track user and administrator activities across workloads in Office 365, which helps with early detection and investigation of security and compliance issues.

Figure 3-4. *Office 365 approach to GDPR*

For healthcare organizations, it is critical to understand the type of personal/patient data they hold and where it resides. Often, we hear that due to compliance standards we cannot move data to the cloud or into anyone else's datacenter. The true question is: How safe is that data in your own datacenter, and how many resources are you willing to commit to protecting that data, as well as how up-to-date are your datacenters and processes relative to the current threat landscape? Many forward-looking organizations have given that responsibility to public cloud providers such as Microsoft and Office 365. There are many Office 365 solutions that can help organizations identify or manage access to personal data:

- Data loss prevention (DLP) in Office and Office 365 can identify over 80 common sensitive data types, including financial, medical, and personally identifiable information. In addition, DLP allows organizations to configure actions to be taken upon identification to protect sensitive information and prevent its accidental disclosure.

- Azure Information Protection (AIP) in Office and Office 365 helps protect data even outside the corporate boundaries. Users can tag documents, such as "Internal," "Confidential," and "External," right within Office clients. Each tag/label has a rights management policy attached to it, which makes sure that the document is protected even if it leaves Office 365. AIP will follow documents wherever they go and will control the documents based on the defined policies.

- Advanced Data Governance uses intelligence and machine-assisted insights to help find, classify, set policies on, and act to manage the lifecycle of the data that is most important to the organization. Advanced Data Governance delivers capabilities such as the following:

  - Proactive policy recommendations and automatic data classifications that allow an organization to take action on data—such as retention and deletion—throughout its lifecycle

  - System default alerts to identify data-governance risks, such as "Unusual volume of file deletion," as well as the ability to create custom alerts by specifying alert-matching conditions and thresholds

  - The ability to apply compliance controls to on-premises data by intelligently filtering and migrating that data to Office 365

- Office 365 eDiscovery search can be used to find text and metadata in content across Office 365 assets—in SharePoint Online, OneDrive for Business, Skype for Business Online, and Exchange Online. In addition, powered by machine-learning technologies, Office 365

Advanced eDiscovery can help identify documents that are relevant to a subject (for example, a compliance investigation) quickly and with better precision than can traditional keyword searches or manual reviews of vast quantities of documents. Advanced eDiscovery leverages machine learning, predictive coding, and text analytics to intelligently reduce the costs and challenges of sorting through large quantities of unstructured data. The eDiscovery process often involves sorting through thousands of email messages, documents, and other data to find the small number of files that may be relevant.

- Customer Lockbox for Office 365 can help meet compliance obligations for explicit data-access authorization during service operations. When a Microsoft service engineer needs access to your data, access control is extended to you so that you can grant final approval for access. Actions taken are logged and accessible to you so that they can be audited.

- Microsoft Cloud App Security is a comprehensive service providing deep visibility, granular controls, and enhanced threat protection for your cloud apps. It identifies more than 15,000 cloud applications in your network—from all devices—and provides risk scoring and ongoing risk assessment and analytics.

Another core requirement of the GDPR is protecting personal data against security threats. The GDPR requires organizations to take appropriate measures to prevent unauthorized access or disclosure and to notify stakeholders in the case of a breach. Today, on average, attacks exist for over 90 days in an environment prior to detection. Current Office 365 features that safeguard data and identify when a data breach occurs include the following:

- Advanced Threat Protection in Exchange Online Protection helps protect email against new, sophisticated malware attacks in real-time. It also allows you to create policies that help prevent your users from accessing malicious attachments or malicious websites linked through email.

- Threat Intelligence helps you proactively uncover and protect against advanced threats in Office 365. Deep insights into threats—insights provided by Microsoft's global presence, the Intelligent Security Graph, and input from cyber threat hunters—help you quickly and effectively enable alerts, dynamic policies, and security solutions.

- Advanced Security Management enables you to identify high-risk and abnormal usage, alerting you to potential breaches. In addition, it allows you to set up activity policies to track and respond to high-risk actions.

- Office 365 audit logs allow you to monitor and track user and administrator activities across workloads in Office 365, which helps with early detection and investigation of security and compliance issues.

- Service encryption with Customer Key: Office 365 announced the availability of service encryption with Customer Key, which can help regulated customers demonstrate additional compliance controls by managing the encryption keys for their Office 365 data.

Today's IT landscape resides in various environments ranging from on-premises to mobile devices to cloud services, and organizations may find that they need to share responsibilities in key areas, such as client and endpoint protection, identity and access management, and application-level controls. An organization will need to assign multiple roles and responsibilities to address all aspects of the GDPR. Regardless of how the organization's governance program is structured, it will be necessary for every team to understand the part it plays in maintaining compliance. Users must be trained to handle data in appropriate ways, security must protect the data without sacrificing productivity, compliance must ensure the controls are in place, IT needs to implement and manage the systems, and business needs to set policies and objectives.

What Is the Urgency?

The General Data Protection Regulation (GDPR) is causing organizations to evaluate their data-processing systems, especially the critical platforms they choose to enable for their workforce. The GDPR is compelling every organization to consider how they will respond to today's security and compliance challenges. It may require significant changes to how your business gathers, uses, and governs data. GDPR goes into effect on May 25, 2018, with broad-reaching implications for EU-based organizations and multinationals around the globe. It's critical to note that the EU GDPR imposes new rules on organizations that offer goods and services to people in the EU, or that collect and analyze data tied to EU residents, no matter where they are located. This means that US-based healthcare entities and organizations defined as controllers or processors of an EU citizen's or resident's healthcare data will be directly affected by GDPR and must be prepared to meet these regulatory requirements. Given how much may be involved, organizations should not wait any longer to prepare. Organizations should review all the privacy and data-management practices now.

Office 365 Security and Compliance Principles

Office 365 is built on the premise that customers own, control, and manage their data stored in Office 365. Microsoft does not use a customer's data for anything other than providing a service that they have subscribed to. As a service provider, Microsoft does not scan customers' email, documents, or teams for advertising or for purposes that are not service related. Microsoft doesn't have access to uploaded content. Like OneDrive for Business and SharePoint Online, customer data stays within the tenant. The Microsoft Security & Trust Center provides more details on the core principles and divides them into four areas, as follows:

1. Built-in Security: It is very important for healthcare providers to maintain ownership of the data all the time, whether the data is sitting in an on-premises datacenter or is in the cloud. Office 365 makes that easy by taking responsibility for keeping data safe and secure while giving full ownership of that data to providers. At the service level, Office 365 uses the defense-in-depth approach to provide physical, logical, and data layers of security features and operational best practices. In addition, Office 365 gives customers enterprise-grade user and admin controls to further secure the environment. Office 365 security consists of these three parts:

a. Built-in security features: Office 365 is a security-hardened service with built-in security features. Providers will benefit from these in-depth security features, which build upon experience gained from two decades of managing online data and significant investment in security infrastructure.

b. Security controls: Office 365 offers security controls that enable providers to customize their security settings. Office 365 is trusted by customers of all sizes across virtually every industry, including highly regulated industries such as healthcare, finance, education, and government. Because Office 365 manages productivity services for such a wide range of industries and geographies, it offers feature choices that customers can control to enhance the security of their data.

c. Scalable security: Office 365 has scalable security processes that allow for independent verification and compliance with industry standards.

2. Continuous Compliance: To help customers with their Office 365–related compliance needs, Microsoft has created a compliance framework that is designed to give customers visibility into Office 365's compliance with global, regional, and industry standards, and also details how customers can control Office 365 services based on compliance needs. Office 365 ensures that compliance expectations are continuously evaluated and incorporated. It is critical for healthcare professionals to ensure that only authorized individuals can access protected health information. Office 365 has capabilities such as data loss prevention, legal hold, email retention, mail policy tips, and Active Directory rights management services. In addition, Office 365 is the first major public cloud service provider that has signed requirements for the Health Insurance Portability and Accountability Act (HIPAA)-Business Associate Agreement with all customers. Office 365 has received authority to operate from a US federal agency under FISMA and has disclosed security measures through the Cloud Security Alliance's public registry.

3. Privacy by Design: When customers entrust their data to Office 365, they remain the sole owner of that data; customers retain the rights, title, and interest in the data you store in Office 365. It is Microsoft's policy to not mine customer data for advertising purposes or use customer data except for purposes consistent with providing you cloud productivity services. *Data privacy* is not allowing personally identifiable information or other sensitive information to be collected, stored, or used without proper consent. With Office 365, the data that organization provides to Microsoft through the use of the service is the organization's data. The organization owns it and controls it. The organization can retrieve that data if it decides to leave the service. The organization remains the sole owner of the data and retains the rights, title, and interest in any data they store in Office 365.

4. Transparent Operations: Moving to a cloud service shouldn't mean losing the ability to know what's going on. With Office 365, it doesn't. Microsoft aims to be transparent in their operations so customers can monitor the state of the service, track issues, and have a historical view of availability.

Office 365 Data Governance

According to a recent Ponemon Institute study (IDC Ponemon Institute, Sponsored by IBM, "Cost of a Data Breach Report," 2016), the average cost of a data breach has risen to $4 million, with costs incurred for litigation, brand or reputation damage, lost sales, and, in some cases, complete business closure. Staying ahead of threats has never been more important. To that end, many organizations have the need to perform surveillance of employee communications. This need stems from internal security and compliance guidelines, or from regulatory bodies such as Financial Industry Regulatory Authority (FINRA). In both cases, failure to have a demonstrable supervision process in place could potentially expose organizations to liability or severe penalties. Today, data is not just about emails and documents; organizations face explosive quantities of complex electronic data across emails, documents, chats, voice and video calls, social media content, and more. Organizations need to supervise employees in order to comply with security and regulatory guidelines and reduce their liability exposure.

Office 365 Advanced Data Governance intelligently eases this information overload by using machine-assisted insights to help you discard ROT: redundant, obsolete, and trivial content. It also efficiently safeguards the high-value content that you need to keep across Exchange Online, SharePoint Online, OneDrive for Business, and Skype for Business. The Office 365 data-governance solution works with a wide array of third-party data sources, with connectors through partners such as the following:

- Social: Twitter, Facebook, LinkedIn, etc.

- Instant messaging: Yahoo Messenger, GoogleTalk, Cisco Jabber, etc.

- Document collaboration: Box, DropBox, Google Drive etc.

- Verticals: SalesForce Chatter, Thomson Reuters, Bloomberg, etc.

- SMS/text messaging: BlackBerry, MobileGuard, etc.

Supervision

The Supervision feature in Office 365 Advanced Data Governance gives compliance officers a practical way to comply with regulations such as HIPAA, FINRA Rule 3110, and SEC Rule 203(e). It lets you define policies about when and how to monitor employee communications and who can monitor them; such communications include email and even Facebook, Twitter, Bloomberg, and more. Organizations can define multiple policies to benefit their needs and to scope whose communications are to be reviewed, under what conditions, and by whom (Figure 3-5).

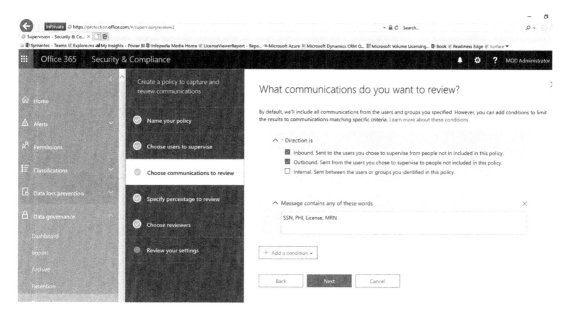

Figure 3-5. *Office 365 Advanced Data Governance, Supervision feature*

Office 365 Advanced eDiscovery

Office 365 Advanced eDiscovery offers a rich set of in-place eDiscovery capabilities to quickly identify relevant data while decreasing costs and risks. Office 365 eDiscovery includes features such as case management, search, hold, analyze, and export to help organizations quickly meet investigative, legal, and regulatory requirements. As a result of the exponential increase in the data, compliance needs are also growing. Spending days or weeks sifting through millions of files to find the few that are relevant is not an option. Office 365 Advanced eDiscovery intelligently uses machine learning, predictive coding, and text analytics to reduce the costs and challenges of sorting through large quantities of unstructured data. Organizations have a need to reduce the volume of data that they must retain, and Office 365 eDiscovery helps in doing so by finding near-duplicate files, reconstructing email threads, and identifying key themes and data relationships.

To configure, go to Security & Compliance Center ➤ Search & investigation ➤ eDiscovery. To discover content, first create a new case and assign users to that case. Once the case is created, administrators can search for a mailbox in Exchange Online or sites in SharePoint Online to put them on hold. Once the item is put on hold, all the subsequent activity will be logged and can be closely monitored. Admins can also search for specific content across all the mailboxes and all the sites and then export the results to the legal team, either internally or externally, for review (Figure 3-6).

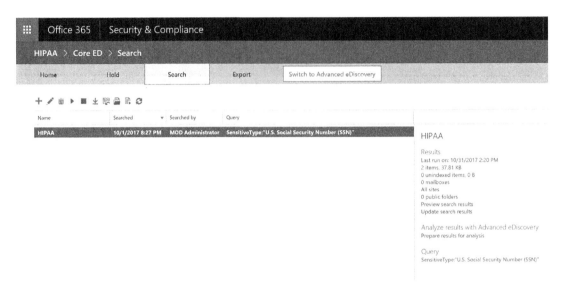

Figure 3-6. *Office 365 eDiscovery Center*

Office 365 Auditing

Office 365 Auditing helps monitor and investigate actions taken on data, intelligently identify risks, contain and respond to threats, and protect valuable intellectual property. Office 365 logs vast numbers of user and admin events based on user activity across services like SharePoint Online, OneDrive for Business, Exchange Online, and Azure Active Directory, which then can be used for investigative purposes. Figure 3-7 shows an example of an audit log search from the Security & Compliance Center.

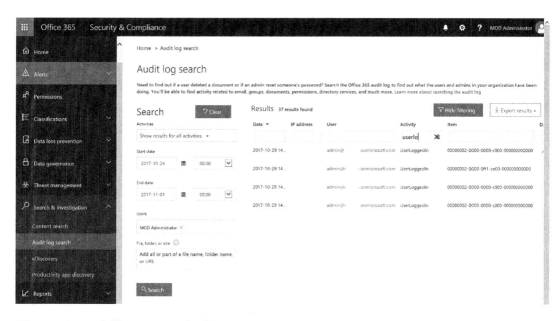

Figure 3-7. Office 365 audit logs

Conclusion

Legacy systems are too inflexible, inefficient, and costly to handle the healthcare-data explosion that has already begun. Managing many point solutions and vendors coupled with the increasing "noise" caused by diverse datasets adds to the complexity of security management and makes it even harder to gain optimal insight into end points and gives even less visibility into the security posture of your entire network. Often, these point solutions don't share any information as they are not integrated, which leads to the most dangerous of these challenges: ineffective responses to threats that grow both in number and sophistication while targeting your organization and your customers. CIOs and IT managers must embrace and quickly adopt a cloud-based strategy and infrastructure to meet the rapidly escalating demands of an increasingly data-driven healthcare industry that is shifting to value-based, patient-centric care and reimbursement models. Having more solutions to deploy and more vendors to manage, with less insight and ineffective threat response, ultimately manifests itself in higher costs of security for Cheif Information Security Officer (CISOs). Organizations that fail to keep up risk being left behind by more agile competitors who move quickly to leverage the cloud's compelling benefits, including significant cost savings and improved management and control of sensitive data and IT assets. An effective security-management solution is not about a single console. Effective security management integrates where it counts, but also offers specialized tools for different functions. Office 365 can help consolidate consoles from many to few while ensuring that specialized teams have the flexibility and freedom to manage their security as per the unique needs of that component, whether it is identity, devices, apps, or infrastructure. Office 365 is a hosted cloud-computing environment that is enterprise class and HIPAA compliant, thus empowering the workforce, care collaboration teams, researchers, and patients with secure, compliant, anytime access using any device.

CHAPTER 4

Telehealth Powered by Office 365

Did you know that the telemedicine concept was invented in the 1960s by NASA? Yes, to monitor astronauts' health from Earth at NASA centers, NASA sent several test flights using animals attached to medical monitoring systems, which sent the animals' biometric data to scientists on Earth via a telemetric link. The focus on the possible limitations of the human body forced NASA to take a technologically focused approach to telemedicine. In situations where a quick return to Earth was not possible, the ability to not only monitor biometric data, but also engage at least rudimentary guided medical treatment by non-physicians, was critical. The same concept applied to remote rural areas where medical help was not available to those who needed it urgently. As we say, necessity is the mother of all invention, and from this necessity was born telehealth. The US military started using telemedicine in the 1980s to combat several natural disasters and conflicts. The American Telemedicine Association (ATA) describes telemedicine as the use of medical information exchanged from one site to another via electronic communications to improve a patient's clinical health status.[1]

Currently, 31 percent of healthcare organizations use video-based telemedicine services, and 34 percent offer remote patient monitoring, according to a KPMG survey conducted by HIMSS Analytics. Expansion plans for these services will drive future use, with another 44 percent of healthcare organizations eyeing video-based telemedicine services and 48 percent planning for remote patient monitoring, the survey of 147 C-suite, IT, and clinical leaders found. By 2018, Kaiser Permanente will perform more virtual visits than in-person office visits. As healthcare evolves toward value-based care

---

[1]Andrew T. Simpson, "A Brief History of NASA's Contributions to Telemedicine," August 16, 2013 (`https://www.nasa.gov/content/a-brief-history-of-nasa-s-contributions-to-telemedicine/`)

N. Dhru, *Office 365 for Healthcare Professionals*, https://doi.org/10.1007/978-1-4842-3549-2_4

incentives rather than the historic fee-for-service reimbursement model, the value of telehealth programs increases multiple times over. Telehealth can be a backbone for healthcare organizations that have very high operating costs, limited clinical staff, and the ambition of providing high-value care more conveniently and in a timely manner to their patients. Patients benefit from having access to leading medical experts miles away from their home who can provide virtual care and personalized real-time treatment while the patients remain in the comfort of their own homes.

Telehealth not only provides convenience to patients but also helps dramatically reduce the treatment cost compared to more expensive inpatient or in-person ambulatory alternatives. Telehealth helps increase quality of care by helping patients better manage chronic disease and addressing critical physician shortages in rural areas. Telehealth efforts have been limited by poor reimbursement for providers, competing demands for capital, and physician skepticism. Some of the new providers are luring patients with more convenient care options that have resulted in mandates for existing providers to manage outcomes and costs in much more efficient ways. The telehealth value proposition is not only limited to providing better care, but has also grown to include capturing higher market share, expanding capacity, and managing costs.

Telehealth services can be divided into three categories: bot agents, live chats, and remote monitoring.

- Bot Agents: This service is an automated service to help answer any preliminary questions from patients via a standard set of clinically based questions, which solicit the necessary information to make a diagnosis, offer treatment recommendations, and, if appropriate, prescribe medication or forward the request to the respective care team. Bots can also help pass critical radiology exam results to remote physicians or pathology tests to remote specialist.

- Live Chats: This service is for real-time interaction with patients through audio or video calls with their care team. Live chats can be used for proactive diagnosis of a disease, a real-time consultation session with remote physicians for a routine follow-up for chronic diseases and prenatal care, getting feedback from multiple physicians from multiple locations for a critical chronic disease, episodic care for seasonal allergies and upper respiratory infections, or behavioral health services.

- Remote Monitoring: This service is for monitoring patients' health via remote consultations, phone apps, or wearable devices that transmit patients' data to providers in a most secure way. Remote monitoring can be used for remote telestroke consultations for neurologists to assess patient symptoms, remote pediatric specialist consultations, or behavioral health and psychiatric assessment. Remote monitoring promotes the use of mobile applications to track specific metrics and promote patient engagement. Patients can upload pictures of their dermatologic conditions that can be reviewed by physicians at a remote location, or diabetic patients can connect a glucometer to their phone that can transmit data to their providers.

Importance of Telehealth

Many healthcare providers are steadily moving to the use of telehealth to reduce emergency room wait times, and they have reported a positive change in providing care onsite at hospitals. The wait time for low-acuity patients in hospitals can vary between two to three-and-a-half hours; with telehealth, all these patients can be seen and treated within 30 to 50 minutes, saving patients time as well as making nurses more efficient in providing care. New York-Presbyterian/Weill Cornell Medical Center has conducted more than 3,000 Telehealth Express Care Service visits to date and has slashed emergency room wait times by more than half because of the Telehealth Express Care virtual visit service. "Our service allows us to streamline care and workflow," said Rahul Sharma, MD, emergency physician-in-chief at New York-Presbyterian/Weill Cornell Medical Center. "Patients seen in our Express Care Service, we remove these patients from the main emergency room so our staff in the main emergency room can focus their attention on more emergent conditions."[2]

Figure 4-1 describes a very high-level flow of telehealth and how it can be operationalized.

---

[2]Bill Siwicki, "New York Hospital Says Telehealth Helped Slash ER Wait Times, Enhance Care," August 17,2017 (http://www.healthcareitnews.com/news/ new-york-hospitals-say-telehealth-helped-slash-er-wait-times-enhance-care)

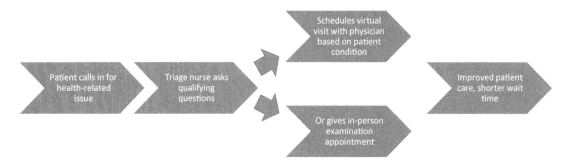

Figure 4-1. *High-level telehalth flow*

No matter which process providers follow, at the root of it patients should get the same or better quality and consistent service irrespective of their location. As shown in the figure, the patient calls the provider call center for a doctor's appointment. The triage nurse asks qualifying questions to make sure the patient is stable for a virtual visit. The triage nurse then schedules either a virtual visit using the teleconferencing service or schedules an in-person visit to the hospital. Only those patients who need in-person care come to the hospital, and the rest gets treated remotely via telehealth service. In either situation, the patient receives treatment from the same physicians who work in the emergency department. Physicians can see more patients via telehealth services, and patients don't have to travel to hospitals for minor symptoms.

Telehealth helps to increase patient reach, retain and acquire new patients, and drive deep relationships with patients by efficiently delivering high-quality care remotely. The "Challenges" section will describe the challenges providers are facing in implementing telehealth even 50 years after its inception.

Challenges

We can classify telehealth challenges in two categories:

1. Technical

2. Non-technical

Technical Challenges

- Securing PHI data: Telehealth, as it is being performed remotely, possesses a big risk of the leakage of patient health information (PHI) if the care team is not careful. Patients can join remotely from public places, which can also expose them to privacy concerns when communicating their personal information out loud in public.

- Single source of truth: Electronic medical record (EMR) systems should be the single source of truth for patient data. Telehealth solutions, if not integrated well with EMR systems, increase the chances of patient data lying around in various systems.

- Availability of internet and computers: The internet is mandatory for telehealth services to reach into rural areas. Computers are not an asset many possess in rural areas, so getting them connected to remote physicians can also be a challenge from their home. The internet is a luxury for many rural villages, so providing telehealth services to them requires significant commitment from both providers and governments.

- Securely sharing information: Videos, audios, texts, and images are sent and received during the telehealth service. Without a secure platform, this information can pose a significant violation of HIPAA and HITRUST regulations.

- Ease of use: Physicians and frontline staff will avoid using technology that seems unwieldy and time-intensive. A higher learning curve will send clinicians away from the telehealth practice. Ease of use is super important for any technology to be popular with doctors and patients.

Non-Technical Challenges

- Physician cross-state license requirements: The lack of licensure portability for physicians and mid-level practitioners is the leading legal barrier to greater adoption of telehealth nationwide. Under most state laws, physicians and mid-level practitioners must be licensed in the state in which they normally practice. Yet, if the patient being treated resides across state lines, a practitioner usually must also be licensed in that state to deliver remote services or meet a possible exception. This creates operational and administrative burdens for physicians who care for patients virtually in multiple states through telehealth.

- Mandatory first physical examination: Rules governing the establishment of a physician–patient relationship are also limiting the growth of telehealth services. In many states, a physician–patient relationship is created once a practitioner has an opportunity to take a patient's medical history and conduct an in-person physical exam. As a result, in most states, physicians are prohibited from remotely prescribing medications without first conducting an in-person physical exam. Additionally, some states require that practitioners conduct in-person exams before providing certain telehealth services to patients who are based in the home or in other settings where a health care provider is not physically present.

- Reimbursement intricacy: Coverage and reimbursement policies by both public and private payers remain obstacles to wider telehealth implementation. Under the Medicare fee-for-service program, there's a limited number of codes that will be reimbursed under the telehealth benefit. Currently, telehealth is covered under the Medicare program only if Medicare beneficiaries present at sites located in rural Health Professional Shortage Areas (HPSAs) or in counties outside Metropolitan Statistical Areas (MSAs). Following updated federal delineations, nearly 100 counties may lose their telehealth benefits, further limiting access to beneficiaries in rural areas.

- Location requirements: Additionally, under the Medicare telehealth benefit, only certain practitioners such as physicians and nurse practitioners may provide services, and they must do so in certain sites such as hospitals or physician offices. Because of these restrictions, reimbursement under the telehealth benefit represents only a minute fraction of the total spending for the Medicare program.

Benefits

Even though telehealth battles significant challenges, it offers several benefits that overshadow these challenges.

- Patient access: Patients frequently encounter long wait times and excessive travel demands for specialty and sub-specialty care. Telehealth reduces travel time and cost for patients. Telehealth also helps minimize patient absenteeism from their work or school. This also helps in acquiring new patients due to convenience provided by provider.

- Cost avoidance: Medical staff shortages contribute to unnecessary patient transfers and avoidable utilization of hospital, care home, and physician resources. Telehealth reduces emergency visits and hospitalizations and prevents unnecessary patient transportation so the patient can receive care in their local nursing homes.[3]

- Patient outreach: Physicians and nurses are unable to meet the demand for their services due to travel requirements. Telehealth creates an opportunity to contract with other provider organizations in need of a specialist coverage. Telehealth generates new revenue in the form of professional billing reimbursement and increases the likelihood of direct referrals when patient transfer is deemed appropriate.

- Extended hours of support: Telehealth with remote monitoring can help increase support hours. Patients can reach a provider any time of the day via teleconferencing and can get quick help on their health condition. Patients don't have to wait for the morning hours for the hospitals to open. They can consult the doctors right from their home even at midnight, which helps improve patient outcomes and patient satisfaction.[4]

---

[3]James R Langabeer, II, Tiffany Champagne-Langabeer, Diaa Alqusairi, Junghyun Kim, Adria Jackson, David Persse, Michael Gonzalez, "Cost-benefit Analysis of Telehealth in Pre-hospital Care," December 5, 2016 (http://journals.sagepub.com/doi/abs/10.1177/1357633X16680541)

[4]Eric Wicklund, "Telemedicine Helps SNFs Improve Patient Care, Curb Hospitalizations," (https://mhealthintelligence.com/news/telemedicine-helps-snfs-improve-patient-care-curb-hospitalizations)

Office 365 for Telehealth

Telehealth is a popular service among technology vendors as they have all realized the potential of the technology to positively impact patient outcomes. These vendors provide a range of telehealth services ranging from simple audio/video conferencing to hospital-wide monitoring systems that include software, hardware, and support. American Well, Avizia, Carena, MDLive, Philips, and Polycom are some of those technology and solution providers in the market. New start-ups have emerged to provide niche mobile and smartwatch solutions. Healthcare providers must consider several options when selecting a telehealth solution, such as clinical use of technology, familiarity with technology of the staff who will use it and support it, hospital priorities and growth strategy, available funds, and so on. Providers have many choices and many point solutions to meet their specific needs. For example, some technologies are more commonly used for episodic disease treatment, either in the acute or ambulatory setting. Others are better suited for disease prevention and disease management and are more often deployed in clinics or patient homes.

Most of the time, healthcare providers will have many similar services inside the organization, as hospitals are usually victims of siloed behavior, and shadow IT is very common. *Shadow IT* means when information technology projects are managed outside of, and without the knowledge of, the IT department. A physician visits a conference or seminar, learns about technology, and asks the hospital to purchase it for his/her department, or a radiologist hears about a different app and advocates its purchase. The provider starts to see the proliferation of specialized apps that solve specific problems, and over time in the environment there will be a collection of apps and solutions that don't talk or work with each other. There will be apps that can help care teams engage with patients while they are at the hospital, but do not provide any way to collaborate remotely. These apps may require clinicians and clients to learn new technology or new ways to interact, and if the apps are complex they will stop using them. From an IT standpoint, it is very difficult to manage and maintain these various apps, which often expose the organization to higher risk with compliance, privacy, and security issues.

Office 365 fits right into this scenario and offers a unified platform of collaboration internally and externally with a highly secure, compliant, and familiar environment. Various services of Office 365 use common productivity tools, which helps clinicians to learn once and use often. These tools (such as Word, PowerPoint, Excel, SharePoint, and Skype) are things they are already using for their day-to-day jobs, so there is no need to spend extra cycles on training with and introducing new apps. IT loves the platform approach, as now they don't need to manage and support various apps; instead, they just need to make the platform available to their users. Anytime there are updates to the underlying platform, the individual solutions automatically benefit from those updates. There's no need to upgrade the apps separately. Because these apps are built on a platform, they share the same backbone, making interoperability very easy. Office 365 also offers all those apps via the cloud and to any device, which makes it easy for clinicians to access their work from anyplace at any time using any device.

Skype for Business (SFB) is one such service and app available via the Office 365 platform. SFB provides communication services for telehealth, telemedicine, telecollaboration, remote patient monitoring, and care coordination. SFB supports instant messaging (IM) and audio and video calls, as well as presence indicators to facilitate communication between clinicians and physicians exchanging critical information. SFB can be integrated with electronic health record systems via its extended APIs; MDLive is a good example of such integration. Many healthcare providers have leveraged third-party partners to build web interfaces with the integration of SFB and other core business needs, such as scheduling appointments, searching for contacts, automated responses based on chat bots, and many other such use cases. SFB provides infrastructure in the Microsoft cloud so providers don't have to worry about setting up infrastructure in their facilities. As long as either patient or clinician has access to the internet and some sort of device, whether it's desktop, laptop, tablet, or phone with browser or app and a camera, they should be able to use the SFB services. All the services in Office 365 including SFB are HIPAA complaint, with encryption end-to-end and continuous monitoring of fraud alerts.

With Office 365 and SFB, it's not just about video or audio conferencing; it's also about providing a high quality of service via high-fidelity video and great voice quality on any device. In a telehealth scenario, patient engagement is key, and making the entire experience very intuitive and easy so that the patient thinks of accessing telehealth when they have a need is critical. SFB also comes in handy in post-discharge cases where patients must report back their health status at regular intervals, so instead of traveling back to the hospital they can report their updates from the comfort of their homes. SFB provides single sign-on capabilities so that clinicians and information workers don't have to re-authenticate to collaborate. Patients, however, will have to authenticate using their credentials to SFB as it is required in order to provide higher security standards.

Configuration

Skype for Business can be accessed from the Office 365 admin portal. Here are the steps to configure SFB in your Office 365 tenant:

1. Sign in to the Office 365 portal from `https://portal.office.com` using your work account.

2. After you sign in, you'll see the Office 365 Admin Center (Figure 4-2).

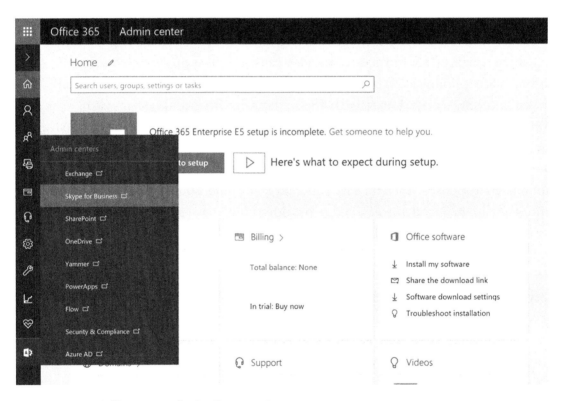

Figure 4-2. *Office 365 Admin Center view*

Click on "Skype for Business," as shown, to log in to SFB portal.

3. Click on the "Users" link from the left-hand menu to get a list of the users (Figure 4-3).

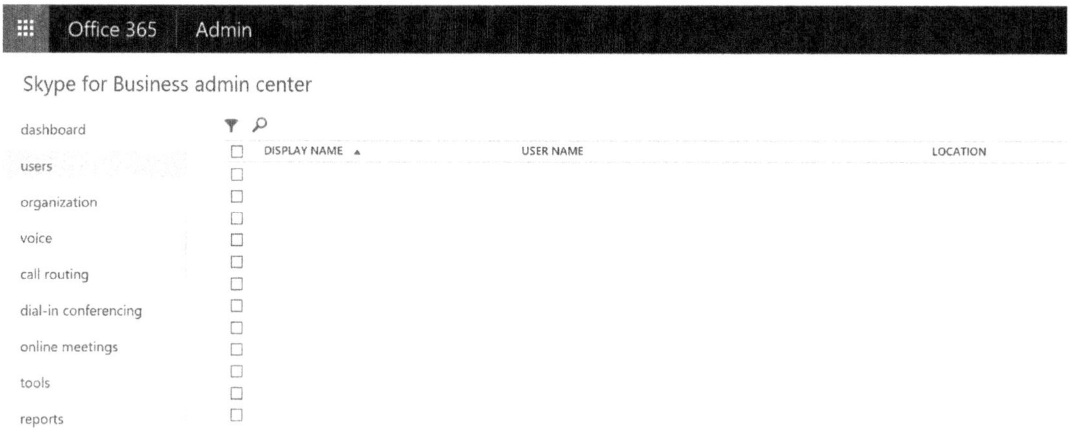

Office 365	Admin

Skype for Business admin center

dashboard
users
organization
voice
call routing
dial-in conferencing
online meetings
tools
reports

DISPLAY NAME ▲   USER NAME   LOCATION

Figure 4-3. *Skype for Business Admin Center view*

You should see all the users you have synced from your on-premises Active Directory on the screen.

4. Choose which users you want to edit for general configuration.

5. Either double-click on the user or select Edit (✎) from the right-side panel.

Option	Details
Audio and HD video	Allow this person to record audio meetings, audio and video meetings, or don't allow them to schedule any meetings (none).
Record conversations and meetings	Choose what this person can record. This option is not available with Skype for Business Basic
For compliance, turn off non-archived features	Choose this option if you're legally required to preserve electronically stored information. Selecting this option turns off features that aren't captured when you have an in-place hold set up in in the Exchange Admin Center. It turns off the following features: <ul><li>File transfer using instant messaging</li><li>Shared OneNote pages</li><li>PowerPoint annotations</li></ul>

6. On the General options page, select or clear the checkbox next to the features you want to change, and then choose "Save."

To configure these settings in bulk, use PowerShell.

7. Configure external communication so that clinicians and information workers can easily collaborate with patients and external physicians (Figure 4-4).

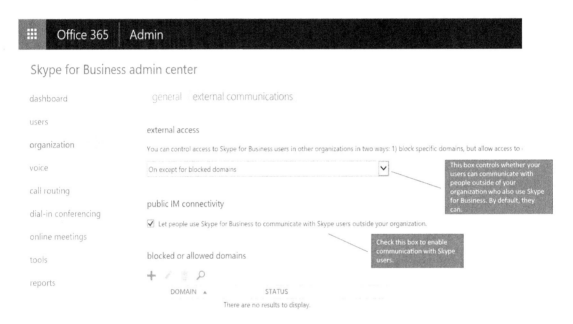

Figure 4-4. *Enable external communication for entire oganization*

IT admins can enable external communication for everyone or can restrict the communication to only certain organizations. The checkbox in the preceding screen will allow Skype users to interact with Skype for Business Online users, which is helpful when patients are using Skype (public free version) to communicate with the care team of a healthcare provider using Skype for Business (enterprise paid version).

8. Configure Presence for entire organization (Figure 4-5).

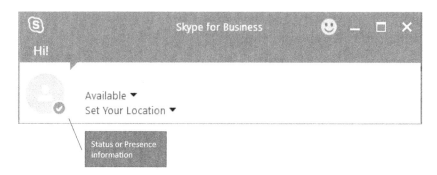

Figure 4-5. *Presence information of a user*

Go to the General tab as in Figure 4-6.

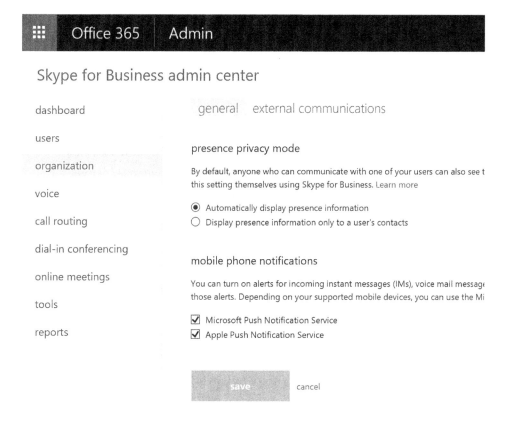

Figure 4-6. *Configure presence for the entire organization*

Under "presence privacy mode," select one of the following settings, and then choose "Save."

Setting	Who can view a user's presence
Automatically display presence information	Any Skype for Business user in your business who has not been added to a person's External or Blocked list will be able to see that person's online presence.
Display presence information only to a user's contacts	Anyone in a person's Contacts list who they have not added to their External or Blocked list. Individuals can override your default settings in their Skype for Business app: Settings ➤ Tools ➤ Options.

The presence indicator is very helpful and identifies if a nurse or clinician is at their desk. The presence indicator saves wait time during the patient transfer from one unit to another and makes sure the required person or team is available at the desired location.

9. Block external access for specified users: After you enable external communication for everyone in your company, you can selectively block external communication for specific individuals using these steps. Select the users whose settings you want to disable and then choose Edit ( ). Choose "External communications" and then clear the options as appropriate:

   - External Skype for Business users: Clear this box if you don't want the user to be able to communicate with Skype for Business users in federated domains.

   - External Skype users: Clear this box if you don't want the user to be able to communicate with people who are using the free Skype app. (Figure 4-7).

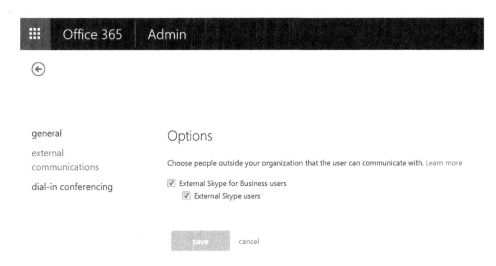

Figure 4-7. Block external sharing for users

10. Download and install Skype for Business app: Organizations will have to figure out a strategy for installing the SFB client on users' computers. Smaller organizations may choose to deploy the SFB client individually on users' computers by the individual users themselves. Larger enterprises may choose to install SFB clients via IT using software-deployment tools such as System Center Configuration Manager. Users can download the Skype for Business app from the app store of their respective devices' vendors, such as iTunes, Google Play Store, or Microsoft App Store.

Chatbot

Telehealth is incomplete without integration with Chatbot. Chatbot is a computer program designed to simulate conversation with human users over the internet using various channels such as Skype or Skype for Business. Imagine a scenario where a patient is calling a healthcare provider's call center to book an appointment or to speak to a nurse about a symptom. For the first one to five minutes the conversation is all based on standard questions and answers, like name, insurance number, reason to call, symptom to report, appointment date and time, and so forth. These are some of the standard Schmitt-Thompson Protocols questions a call center agent or triaging nurse will ask, as these are industry-standard questions thoroughly reviewed by a panel of nurse consultants, medical directors, primary-care providers, specialists, and ER doctors. This is where Chatbot can help and take the burden off of call center agents or triaging nurses.

The patient logs into their Skype app, finds a chatbot provided by their healthcare provider, and starts asking questions. The chatbot starts answering those questions, leveraging the well-documented Schmitt-Thompson Protocol questions and answers. By the time the call reaches a triaging nurse, all generic questions have already been answered by the chatbot, and now the triaging nurse will only have to ask very specific questions. A training nurse can see the conversation history either via the same chatbot interface or via an integrated interface to their existing call-logging system. Chatbots are capable of receiving and sending information from other line-of-business applications, so integration with existing systems should be straightforward. Chatbots can help reduce the time triaging nurses spend asking and answering those generic questions. This is a huge productivity boost for triaging nurses, and all healthcare providers should invest in such technology.

Creating a chatbot in Skype for Business is easy. It requires third-party vendors to develop a specific chatbot for the healthcare provider. Microsoft has developed a chatbot for their healthcare customers; you can find out more about it at `https://www.healthvault.com/en-us/health-bot/`. Skype for Business also provides a bot framework that can be leveraged for creating and deploying a chatbot within an enterprise; more details can be found at `https://msdn.microsoft.com/en-us/skype/skype-for-business-bot-framework/docs/overview`.

Dial-in or PSTN Conferencing

In healthcare environments where clinicians are always on the move, sitting at a desk to join meetings or conferences is sometimes just not possible. They need to be able to dial in to the meeting using their phones or to have the conferencing system call them and add them to the meeting with one simple click. Skype for Business includes the dial-in conferencing feature for just this situation. Clinicians or information workers can call into Skype for Business meetings using a phone instead of using the Skype for Business app on a mobile device or PC.

Skype for Business also allows users to join the audio portion of an SFB conference call (i.e., participants) by having the SFB online call *out* to whatever number the user specifies. This could be their cell phone, desk phone, or any manually specified phone number, provided the user is enabled for it.

Skype for Business users can also set up the call-forwarding option so that SFB knows when to forward an incoming call if not picked up in under 60 seconds. Call forwarding lets you choose how you want Skype for Business to handle incoming calls when you're away from your work phone, such as when nurses are visiting patients, or when you want someone else to take your calls. Figure 4-8 shows where to change the call-forwarding settings in the Skype for Business client.

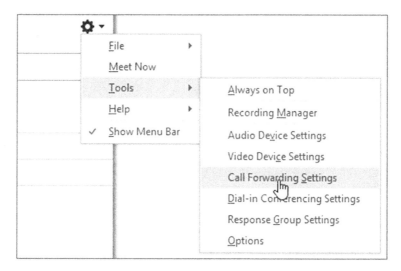

Figure 4-8. *Setting up call forwarding*

Meeting Broadcast

Skype Meeting Broadcast is a feature of Skype for Business Online and Office 365 that enables you to schedule, produce, and broadcast meetings or events to online audiences of up to 10,000 attendees. This feature is useful when, for instance, a nurse manager wants to provide educational content or updated information in one-to-many settings. Nurses can be in any facility, within or outside of the country, but can still join the conference using any device. Care teams can use the Meeting Broadcast feature to educate patients in the community about common diseases and how to counter them, or to involve physicians from different disciplines and hospitals for a patient case.

The Skype for Business admin will have to enable Meeting Broadcast from the Office 365 Admin Center, as shown in the following steps:

1. Sign in with your Office 365 global admin account at
   `https://portal.office.com/adminportal/home`.

2. In the Office 365 Admin Center, go to Admin Centers ➤ Skype for Business.

3. Go to Skype for Business Admin Center ➤ Online Meetings ➤ Broadcast Meetings. Then, click "Enable Skype Meeting Broadcast."

Once Meeting Broadcast is enabled, browse to `https://portal.broadcast.skype.com`, sign in using your work account, click on "New meeting," and fill in the date and time and so forth to schedule a meeting broadcast (Figure 4-9).

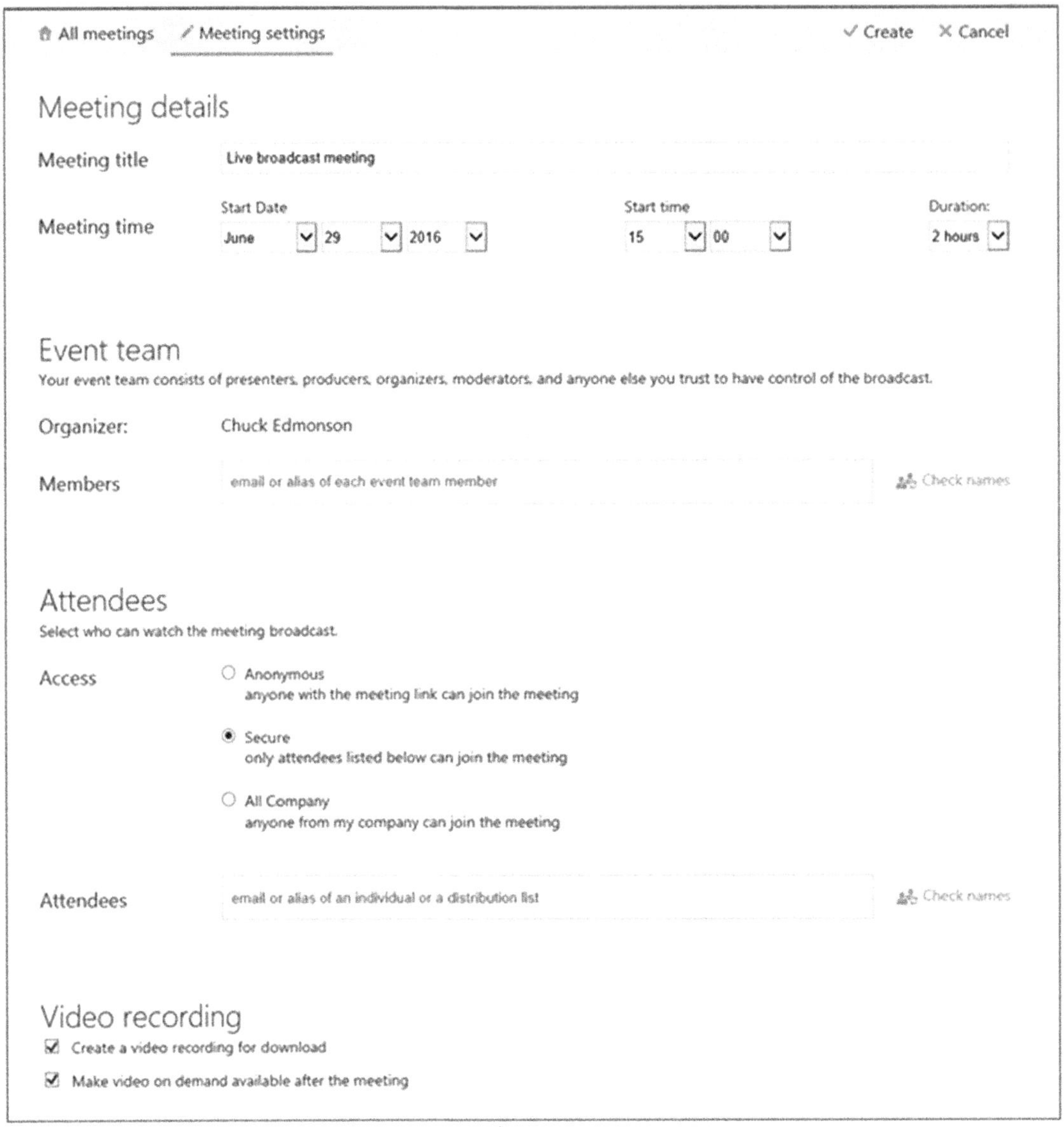

Figure 4-9. *Setting up a meeting broadcast*

Security and Compliance

As we know, compliance and security are two fundamental pillars of anything that happens within the healthcare industry. SFB and Office 365 follow all the needed compliance standards (HIPAA, HITRUST) and provide end-to-end security for the environment. Office 365 and SFB make sure that PHI is only accessed after login and all information is encrypted both at rest and in transit. Patient privacy is the topmost concern for any healthcare provider, and in telehealth it becomes even more important, as services can be delivered via smartphones, mobile applications, tablets, computers, and other methods. Making telehealth accessible in this way also makes it very difficult for providers to follow security standards and meet HIPAA and other regulations, but Office 365 can help in this scenario.

Telehealth can contribute to the accumulation of a large volume of regulated health information across different mediums (audio, video, text, and image). Managing and storing such large datasets and integrating this information, in its various mediums, into electronic medical records can create compliance challenges under HIPAA (such as complying with medical-record access and accounting requirements, preserving the integrity of PHI, and safeguarding security). Providers who practice telehealth across state lines must also contend with multiple, and sometimes very different, state and federal privacy requirements that present a challenge. If you prefer to not preserve conversations and meeting recordings as well as to not allow users to do file transfers, share OneNote pages, or do PowerPoint annotations, then SFB can be configured in this manner. Figure 4-10 shows how to disable those features.

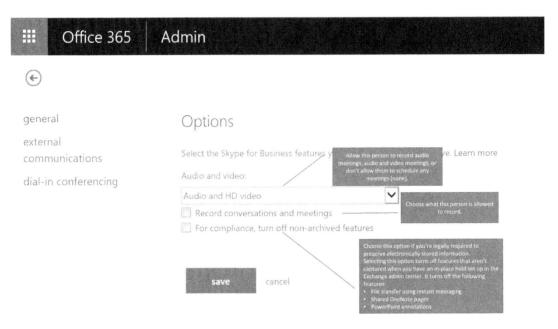

Figure 4-10. *Turn off non-archived features*

Go to Office 365 portal ➤ Sign in using work account ➤ From the Admin Center select "Skype for Business" ➤ Choose users and click on Edit or use PowerShell for bulk update.

Any breach in patient health information can result in legal action, and steps must be taken to inform the subject whose privacy has been violated, as well as to report the breach to a long list of federal, state, and local authorities, sometimes including the media. To protect against situations like this, SFB has designed the features, and it is up to the implementer—in this case the healthcare provider—to configure the platform accordingly. Setting up these rules as shown in Figure 4-10 can prevent video, voice, screens, chat, or IM from being shared outside of corporate walls. In the event where information must be sent outside to external physicians or clinicians for legitimate reasons, Office 365 offers a file-sharing platform known as SharePoint Online or OneDrive for Business. Through SharePoint Online or OneDrive for Business, providers can securely share information externally by rights protecting the file and running data leak prevention (DLP) policies before sharing externally. Securely sharing files externally is discussed in detail in Chapter 7, "Personal Health Record External Sharing Securely."

Conditional Access for Skype for Business

Your organization may have requirements where users should not be able to access Skype for Business while not at work. In healthcare, there are specific regulations that don't allow clinicians to have access to office tools from home. It is very important to note that Skype for Business Online is a cloud-based solution, so without configuring conditional access, users can access it from anywhere using any device by entering their work account credentials. This can create conflicts with security and regulation policies; hence, configuring a conditional access policy is crucial.

Figure 4-11 shows the condition flow to verify if a user's device is compliant and thus to allow the user to access SFB from that device.

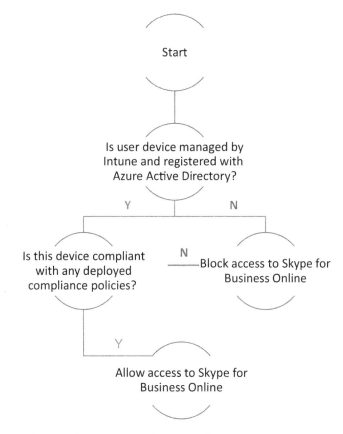

Figure 4-11. *Conditional access verification flow*

For configuring conditional access policy for Skype for Business Online, follow the steps described in this article: `https://technet.microsoft.com/en-us/library/mt712706.aspx?f=255&MSPPError=-2147217396`.

Telehealth Use Case

In this section, we will review a sample use case that can be hypothetically converted into a telehealth session. The provider can customize this use case based on their needs, but it should give them a good idea of how to convert an existing process to a telehealth service. This use case is about pediatric telehealth. Clinical staff shortages and patient-access barriers are two of the primary drivers of telehealth adoption for pediatric services. Approximately one-third of children must travel 40 miles or more to receive care from a pediatric sub-specialist, and the average wait time for their appointments ranges between five weeks and three months.[5]

In a study by UC–Davis, 83 percent of parents with children requiring specialist care reported travel time exceeding one hour, and 40 percent missed work to accommodate their child's appointment.[6] Additionally, the mean age of pediatric sub-specialists exceeds 50 years, and an aging workforce is likely to exacerbate these provider shortages and patient-access issues. Pediatric telehealth can be used for virtual interactions between providers, patients under the age of 18, and their parents or caregivers. Pediatric telehealth can help facilitate specialist consultations, diagnosis and treatment, and patient education. Pediatric telehealth can be used for both acute

---

[5]Gage, D., "America's Children Need Access to Pediatric Subspecialists," *American Academy of Pediatrics*, accessed September 29, 2015; available at: `http://www2.aap.org/visit/Sec5203FactSheet.pdf`

[6]James P. Marcin, et al., "Using Telemedicine to Provide Pediatric Subspecialty Care to Children with Special Health Care Needs in an Underserved Rural Community," *Pediatrics*, Vol. 113, No. 1(2004): 1–6.

and chronic conditions and can be targeted to medically underserved rural and inner-city populations. Pediatric telehealth can support conditions such as asthma, diabetes, cardiac conditions, epilepsy, and mental health disorders. The equipment and resources required for pediatric telehealth depend on the types of services offered and may include videoconference platforms and web cameras, mobile apps, smartphones or tablets, wearable patient monitors, and web-based patient portals or peer-networking websites. At a minimum, these devices must sustain the audio and visual capabilities necessary to conduct remote patient assessment and provider communication.

Imagine a scenario where after the implementation of pediatric telehealth, the parent of a patient walks up to the computer and browses a website or opens an app from their mobile phone. This website or mobile app (integrated with Skype consumer version) is developed and maintained by the provider for their patient for telehealth use. The parent clicks an "I need help" button on the interface (we will call this an interface, but this means either a website page or a page in a mobile app), and a chat window will open. Skype for Business Online and Skype consumer version both support the development and deployment of custom chatbots. The automated chatbot greets the parent and asks how he/she can help. The conversation could go as shown in Figure 4-12.

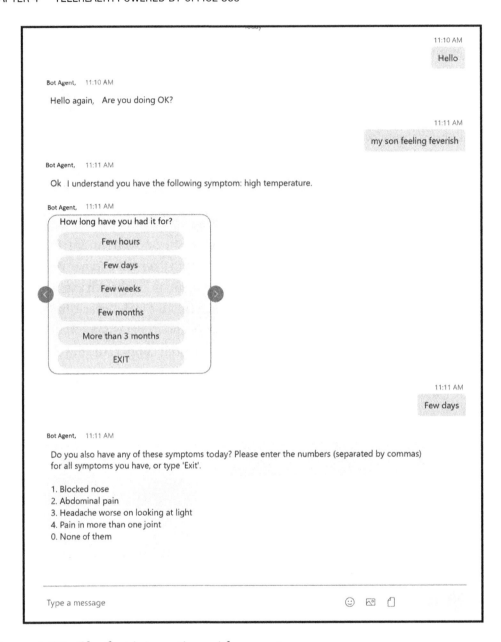

Figure 4-12. *Chatbot interacting with parent*

After standard questions and answers, the bot agent may decide to pass the request to a triage nurse in the same interface or to schedule an appointment with the doctor either in person or virtually. Because the bot knows who you are based on your profile information from the app, it knows who your primary-care physician is and can check the appointment availability of that physician to set up the consultation accordingly.

Once the appointment is scheduled and the invitation for that appointment is sent to both physician and patient, the app can remind the patient and physician via text or alert notification 15 minutes prior to the appointment time. At the appointment time, assuming the consultation is virtual, both patient and physician can sit in front of their screens—it could be a PC or a mobile phone with app—to start the conversation. The patient could be using Skype consumer version and the physician could be using Skype for Business, as users can communicate across those two apps (Figure 4-13).

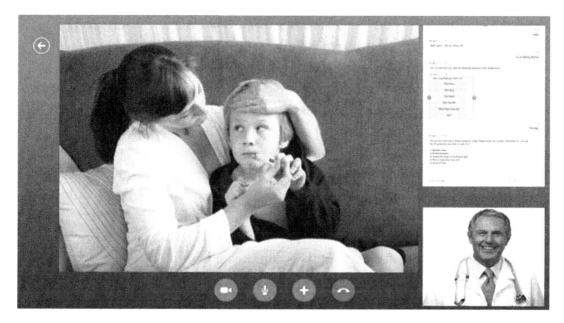

Figure 4-13. *Pediatric telehealth session in progress*

The physician might already have all the patient's vitals prior to the consultation if the patient is wearing a remote monitoring device, smart watch, or something like that. The app can resurface that information in the same screen as the chat interface so that doctors have all the vital information of a patient. Below screen shows how Skype can be integrated into the EMR system so that doctors can have a 360-degree view of the patient and all information can be stored within the EMR during the telehealth virtual session.

In the event where the EMR system is not fully integrated with the telehealth system, the doctor can keep taking notes within the same custom app, which can be linked to the Office 365 OneNote service. This way all the information is synced back to the EMR system once the consultation is over. If desired, the entire virtual conversation can be recorded for future discovery purposes. These recordings can be saved in the same space as the patient's OneNote, either in OneDrive or SharePoint.

Conclusion

Reducing healthcare costs while improving patient outcomes is a primary concern worldwide. By 2020, healthcare will consume 10.5 percent of world gross domestic product (GDP). Demand for healthcare services will only increase in the future given population growth, longer lifespans, the rise of chronic disease, clinician shortages, strained budgets, and recent natural disasters. Digital technologies are transforming the way consumers work, shop, and socialize. Healthcare providers are beginning to deploy digital tools to better understand and serve their patients, especially those with the greatest health needs who typically incur the highest costs. Telehealth has been instrumental in allowing those who are limited and restricted to receive the medical attention of medical professionals. Telehealth enhances the patient–physician relationship by enabling providers to offer better education and personalized feedback remotely. The ability to consult virtually and collaborate at a distance makes caregivers more productive as well as reaches underserved patient populations to reduce delays that can result in costly or catastrophic outcomes. Physicians can gain quicker access to other professionals remotely and can share digital images, audio files of heartbeats, and fetal movements in seconds via a telehealth platform. Telehealth doesn't replace the direct, in-person connection between patient and providers, but it helps increase patient and physician satisfaction while providing better patient outcomes.[7] Telehealth and other digital technologies have started playing a crucial role in hospital exam rooms, board rooms, and waiting rooms. Telehealth is constantly evolving, and there are many technology-solution providers who are providing high-value services, but it still faces the non-technical challenges described earlier. Benefits provided by telehealth overshadow the challenges it poses.

Leveraging Skype for Business as a technology for telehealth services will not only help providers increase their return on investment but will also make providers more secure and compliant. Skype or Skype for Business, with their very familiar user interface and ease of operation, make it a viable technology for every telehealth setup. The Skype for Business platform makes virtual health solutions accessible and customizable, obviating the need to purchase, learn, and maintain expensive dedicated apps to reduce gaps in the health service provided by healthcare providers. Telehealth in its true sense helps providers and hospitals digitally transform their business and services globally.

---

[7]Andrew Broderick and David Lindeman, The Commonwealth Fund, Case Studies in Telehealth Adoption, January 2013.

CHAPTER 5

Innovations in Tumor Board Reviews

A tumor board review (TBR) is a treatment planning approach in which many doctors who are experts in different medical specialties, and often are from different hospitals, review and discuss the medical condition and treatment options of a patient. In many countries, the tumor board review is an important phase in the multidisciplinary oncological care pathway. In cancer treatment, a tumor board review may include a medical oncologist (who provides cancer treatment with drugs), a surgical oncologist (who provides cancer treatment with surgery), and a radiation oncologist (who provides cancer treatment with radiation). It is also called a multidisciplinary opinion. A tumor board is a regularly scheduled (typically weekly) meeting where cancer cases are discussed in a comprehensive manner. There is typically a pathologist present to review biopsy and surgical specimens, with the microscopic pictures projected on a large screen, as well as a radiologist to review pertinent scans. The tumor board functions as a comprehensive second opinion and allows specialists to have input on how cancer cases should be treated, thereby creating a type of community standard. The recommendations are not binding but are very helpful in tough cases. Some tumor boards are limited to one kind of cancer. Most commonly, these are for breast and lung cancer because of the frequency of cases. Others are general tumor boards where cases requiring complicated treatment decisions are reviewed.

The boards function in several formats, including the following:

- As part of a regularly held, multidisciplinary clinic where specialists personally evaluate patients, then meet as a board to discuss each case (they also may review cases requested by community-based clinicians)

- As stand-alone meetings to review cases, complete with diagnostic imaging, biopsy findings, and the patients' medical histories

© Nidhish Dhru 2018
N. Dhru, *Office 365 for Healthcare Professionals*, https://doi.org/10.1007/978-1-4842-3549-2_5

- As virtual meetings with visual and audio communication between multiple locations

Multidisciplinary tumor boards sometimes give their treatment recommendations directly to the patient; in all other cases, they speak to the requesting physician. Patients may then choose where to be treated. Physicians post patient imaging scans and other data on the hosting software. All participants simultaneously see on-screen views as clearly as if in their own clinic.

The main output of a tumor board review is a report containing the collective findings, conclusions, and recommendations for the further treatment of the patient. This may also include the recommendation to include a patient in a clinical research trial. Tumor board review meetings also serve as a platform for sharing the latest guidelines, developments, and insights in the diagnosis and treatment of the specific cancer type. The sharing of knowledge is seen as a valuable asset.

Table 5-1 outlines the roles present during the TBR process.

Table 5-1. *Roles During Tumor Board Review*

Role	Function
Radiologist	Review of medical images
Pathologist	Review of biopsies
Oncologist	Chemotherapy
Radiotherapist	Radiotherapy
Specialized nurse	Counseling, main contact person
Plastic surgeon	Plastic surgery
Case manager	Management of overall case
Psychologists	Counseling on psychological stress
Surgical oncologist	Surgical management of tumors

Although many community hospitals have local tumor boards that review all types of cases, many providers, particularly in rural areas and smaller institutions, still lack access to tumor boards specializing in a particular type of cancer (e.g., breast, gastrointestinal, hematologic cancers). During TBR discussions, physicians can explain minimally invasive procedures and offer insight into when interventional care is the safest and most effective form of treatment. Other times, the best treatment is a combination of two specialties—such as surgeons and radiation oncologists collaborating to provide optimal care. In either case, tumor board discussions allow physicians to acknowledge the benefits and setbacks of a variety of procedures, giving patients a wider array of options than if the oncologist had simply made a decision on his or her own.

TBR Process Flow

High-level patient-treatment phases are shown in Figure 5-1.

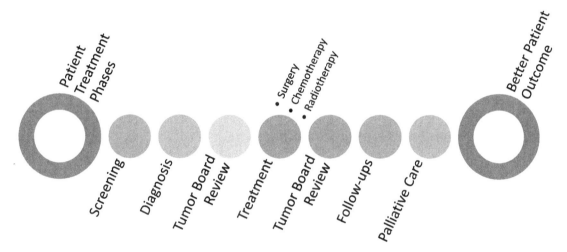

Figure 5-1. *Patient-treatment phases*

The patient usually goes through the phases described. The physician recommends a screening after seeing the patient's health condition. After the screening is done, a specialist such as a radiologist or pathologist views the results and provides feedback to the physician. Based on the results and feedback from the specialist, the physician may decide to take the patient's case through tumor board review. The outcome of the tumor board review guides the physician on a potential path to treatment. Treatment may include surgery, chemotherapy, radiotherapy, and so forth. After treatment, the physician may still review the patient's health with the tumor board. The tumor board can recommend a specific follow-up procedure for ongoing treatment. Palliative care continues throughout the continuum of care and is focused on treating the patient's symptoms.

Figure 5-2 describes the tumor board review process in detail.

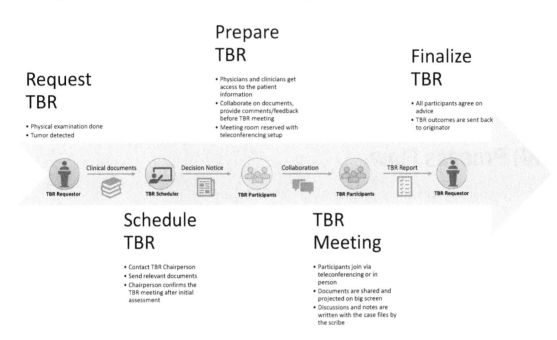

Figure 5-2. *Tumor board review process flow*

The TBR process has five distinct steps, and each one has its own owner and list of participants based on their role in the process as well as on their role in the organization. Each participant has their own rights and duties in this process and is responsible for driving the process forward with clarity and full ownership.

Table 5-2 shows the different participants in the TBR process, their roles, and their responsibility in each phase.

Table 5-2. *Participants During Tumor Board Review*

Participant	Description
TBR Requestor	Participant (healthcare professional, e.g., gastroenterologist) who initiates the TBR request. Submits the request and the related supporting documents
TBR Scheduler	Participant responsible for the scheduling of the tumor board review by providing one of the timeslots for the requested TBR
TBR Preparator	Any participant that is part of the tumor board and involved in the review process
TBR Reporter	A participant (usually a healthcare professional) who writes down the conclusions of the tumor board review
TBR Finalizer	A participant who validates the preliminary tumor board review report

Request TBR: TBR requestor, who is usually the primary physician, may decide to present the case to the tumor board for review if the patient meets the criteria of a certain tumor board review. In this step, clinical documents such as documents, images, or reports that have led to the diagnosis of the patient will have to be sent to the review board. TBR requestor provides other information, such as reason for TBR, with short descriptions to the review board.

Schedule TBR: TBR scheduler, who can be the chairperson of the TBR or a medical secretary, reads the request for admission to the TBR and checks the documents and criteria for the TBR. The scheduler uses the information that has been sent for the assessment and decides whether, and when, the case will be presented in one of the next TBR meetings. A decision notice is sent back to the requestor with the information about when and where the TBR meeting will be held. A decision notice is created for each patient, as they can be presented at a different time and date. A decision notice can act like a reference point for the upcoming TBR meeting.

Prepare TBR: In this step, the TBR preparator consolidates all the information related to the TBR and distributes it to the TBR participants. Participants at this point can start asking questions and start adding more information to the case. Participants can also ask for more information from the requestor related to the case. This step is the beginning of the review process where participants start collaborating, even before the TBR meeting takes place. This steps also makes sure that participants are familiar with the case before coming to the meeting.

TBR Meeting: In this step, all the TBR members convene and discuss the cases that have been scheduled, using all relevant information that has been gathered by the team members. The discussion between members leads to a consensus-based diagnosis and a recommendation for the further treatment of the patient. A TBR report is generated as the output of the findings and recommendations by a committee, and will be approved by all the participants.

Finalize TBR: In this final step, the TBR report is shared with the TBR requestor with the relevant patient information, the original request of the requestor, and the information of the TBR report. The TBR report may vary between the specific tumor boards. The finalized TBR report can also be shared with the general physician of the patient or any other designated party.

TBR Advantages

- After TBR feedback, patients have higher confidence in the treatment plan as the case was reviewed and discussed at length by a multidisciplinary team instead of just one doctor.

- After the TBR feedback, the patient can be sent back to the hospital nearest to home, where friends and family can give more care and provide assistance. With TBR, knowledge is not limited to one facility or hospital; knowledge of new experiments and evolving treatments can be spread to the smallest town and the biggest city.

- Small-town hospitals can refer patients to larger hospitals based on the findings from the TBR to leverage broader expertise and more sophisticated instruments for better patient care.

- A TBR also helps in expediting patient care, which otherwise might take weeks of waiting to be seen by many specialists for a treatment. All specialists related to that treatment are present in the TBR and make the decision on treatment. This also increases the likelihood of faster patient healing.

- A TBR also increases the chances that the patient will be offered participation in a clinical trial.

- A TBR helps in providing more personalized care for a patient dealing with rare diseases. A TBR also can be useful for finding new interpretations of pathologic or imaging studies that could influence treatment recommendations.

- Sometimes after the TBR, a patient's physician changes the treatment approach as more specialists comment on the treatment. This results in accurate and more effective treatment for the patient, which increases patient satisfaction and reduces readmission rate.

- A TBR gives a physician a range of different treatment options, which helps in deciding the best suitable treatment for the patient. This is helpful as patients with cancer often have a unique set of comorbidities that make undergoing traditional surgery risky.

- A TBR helps in the ongoing education process of oncologists, surgeons, and other specialists.

- A TBR helps interventional radiologists stay in the forefront of the cancer care. New treatments, techniques, and clinical trials are often discussed in TBRs, giving interventional radiologists a glimpse into cutting-edge cancer research and advancements in the medical field. More-educated interventional staff helps improve patient care and patient satisfaction and, eventually, allows hospitals to extend their offerings into more advanced treatments.

- New research opportunities can be discovered during the TBR process. These new research opportunities may someday help reduce the treatment costs, improve patient care, and reduce readmission rates.

- A TBR not only helps educate the immediate staff but also helps educate the staff at hospitals and care centers where the patient will be admitted. Nurses can learn the latest treatments and new ways of engaging with patients. Physicians are educated to the roles of the so-called paraprofessionals so that all hospital and community resources are being used to the patient's advantage.[1]

---

[1]"The Value of Multidisciplinary Tumor Boards in Cancer Care," August 2017 (https://www.navify.com/wp-content/uploads/2017/08/Value-of-Tumor-Boards-in-Cancer-Care.pdf)

TBR Challenges

- It is important that the right doctor is in the review board, otherwise the meeting will have no positive outcome. Making reviews available remotely not only increases the chances of the right doctor's being available but also broadens the reach to doctors across states and nations.

- Multidisciplinary clinics with tumor boards are resource-intensive and challenging for scheduling physician's time, which may contribute to the overall cost of the TBR.

- One common platform is required to manage all the relevant documents associated with the TBR; it should have the ability for all participants to share and provide feedback in one single place. A disjointed experience and messed-up version of the documents distracts from the real purpose of the meeting.

- The TBR requestor and TBR scheduler have to go through the cumbersome process of creating a document package for the TBR meeting. Images and documents (because of their size) sometimes need to be sent via CD or DVD. The physical copy of this data sometimes loses its relationship with the electronic record, and it can be difficult to trace it back to the right patient for the right TBR. This is a time-consuming and human error–prone process and needs a common platform for the creation and sharing of content for the TBR.[2]

- The TBR scheduler plays a very important role in scheduling the TBR meeting, matching the right patient's case with the right TBR meeting, finding out the availability of the needed physicians and specialists, finding out if the right equipment is available during the time of the TBR meeting, and moving cases around based on the time available and number of cases to review. All these activities take time to coordinate by calling/emailing individuals for their availability, making re-arrangements, and so forth. There is also a need to have

---

[2]"Tumor Board Workflow Challenges in Preparation, Presentation and Documentation," July 2017 (https://www.navify.com/wp-content/uploads/2017/09/Tumor-board-workflow-challenges-in-preparation-presentation-and-documentation.pdf)

one single consolidated place where the TBR scheduler can see the status of all TBRs and then decide the case outcomes based on that.

- Making sure the right participants have the right information before and after the meeting is key. Radiologists should be able to securely view CT scans, X-ray images, and endoscopic images before the TBR meeting. Making sure those images do not leave the hospital boundaries requires sophisticated tools. Without a common platform, keeping all the required documents in one single place is a challenge and creates confusion for the participants regarding what is the single source of truth.

- As a result of a lack of information of patient case during the TBR meeting, sometimes patients that were scheduled cannot be discussed. Sometimes patients are coming from different hospitals. A lack of information regarding their health history can delay the process, as without knowing the full history, the board cannot make a final recommendation. Meeting notes should be captured accurately to make sure patient case has all the related information on past reviews. After the meeting, those notes are consolidated, and once again the TBR scheduler has to send that to participants, who then validate those notes and confirm or provide modifications. This creates extra cycles and delays the final TBR report's completion.

Tools and Services That Can Help

As previously discussed, it is very important to make it easy for participants to join the review board meetings from anywhere using any device. Collaboration is the fundamental component for any TBR to be successful. The challenges described the preceding section are real challenges every TBR member faces each day. The following section will help address some of the challenges via modern tools and technologies, but again, for any system to be successful its users should adopt that new technology with a growth mindset. Before we go too deep into how this technology will help improve the TBR process, let's spend some time understanding the technology itself.

Microsoft Teams Overview

Office 365 offers a collaboration toolset named Microsoft Teams that can be leveraged in its totality to help improve the TBR process. MS Teams conglomerates different services into one single umbrella with a modern intuitive user interface. This tool can be installed on local computers or accessed via internet/mobile devices, thus removing accessibility barriers. Microsoft Teams is a messaging app for teams where all conversations, meetings, files, and notes can be accessed by everyone, all in one place. Figure 5-3 shows some of the features of Microsoft Teams.

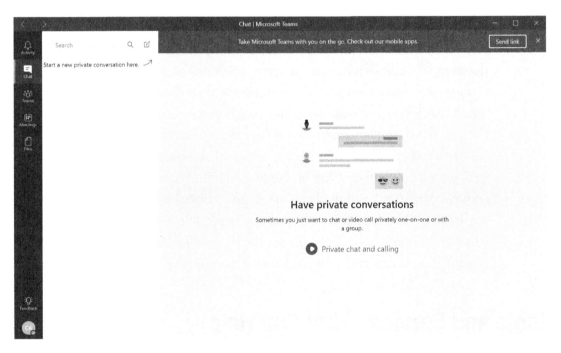

Figure 5-3. *Microsoft Teams' main screen*

Messaging: Microsoft Teams offers one-on-one or group chat experiences. It also offers a persistent chat experience where the prior chat of other team members is retained, and when a new member joins the team, he or she can go through the previous chat history of the team. Team conversations are visible to the entire team, and there is also a functionality to do private one-on-one chats with individual team members. Microsoft Teams also offers voice and video conferencing, so anyone from the team can start an audio or video call that the entire team can join from anywhere using any device.

One place for collaboration: Microsoft Teams brings together an entire productivity suite under one single user interface. Word, Excel, PowerPoint, SharePoint, OneNote, Planner, Power BI, and Delve are all built into Microsoft Teams so the team can have all the information and tools they need for the TBR review process. It also offers searchability across various teams that you are part of, so one quick search can get you results from a similar TBR review. Teams enables teams to get on a call using voice and video from the same interface. Participants can take notes and share images in the call from the same Teams space.

Unique for each team: Microsoft Teams can be customized for each team or for each TBR meeting. Teams can add additional content via the tabs/apps section shown in Figure 5-4 to bring more content and information for a specific team or TBR meeting.

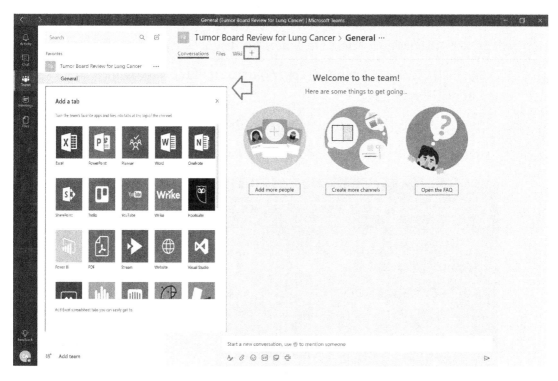

Figure 5-4. *Microsoft Teams, available tabs*

These tabs can also be extended for line-of-business apps as Microsoft Teams provides an open API framework for integration.

Highly secure collaboration: Microsoft Teams provides the advanced security and compliance capabilities that any healthcare provider demands. All the data is encrypted in transit and at rest. Microsoft Teams also supports key compliance standards, including EU Model Clauses, ISO 27001, SOC 2, HIPAA, and more. Teams works on the same framework as Office 365 that makes it possible to restrict permission for who can view and contribute to the content.

Accessible anywhere: Microsoft Teams is available on tablets, phones, and the web so everyone who is part of the review board can access MS Teams anywhere, anytime, using any device. This will help ensure all participants are available at a given time no matter where they are physically located.

Configure Microsoft Teams in Office 365

Here are the steps to configure Microsoft Teams inside the Office 365 tenant:

1. Sign in to Office 365 tenant (`https://portal.office.com`) with your work account.

2. Choose "Admin" to go to the Office 365 Admin Center.

3. Go to Settings ➤ Services & add-ins, as shown in Figure 5-5.

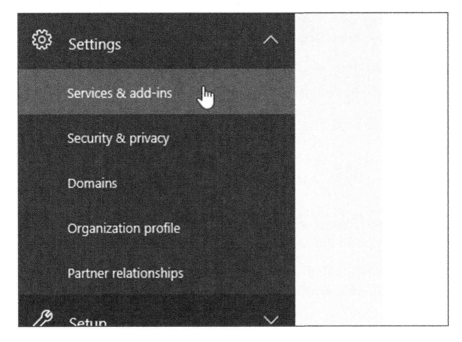

Figure 5-5. *Microsoft Teams, Office 365 admin add-ins*

4. On the Services & Add-ins page, select "Microsoft Teams,"
   as shown in Figure 5-6.

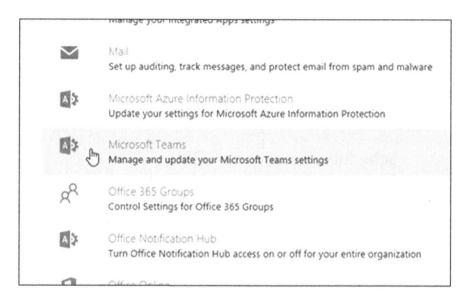

Figure 5-6. *Office 365 ➤ Microsoft Teams selection*

5. On the Microsoft Teams Settings page that opens, click or tap
   the toggle next to "Turn Microsoft Teams on or off for your entire
   organization" to *On* to turn on Teams for your organization, and
   then choose "Save." If you don't want to allow Microsoft Teams in
   your organization, click or tap to switch the toggle to Off.

MS Teams and TBR Process Flow

In this section, we will review a TBR process flow that uses improved technology like
MS Teams. Figure 5-7 shows the MS Teams and TBR process flow:

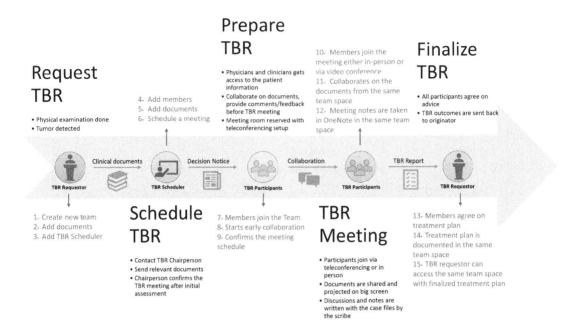

Figure 5-7. *MS Teams and TBR process flow*

This diagram overlays the new process in red for each phase. Screening, diagnosis, treatment, and aftercare of oncological patients require the cooperation of a multidisciplinary team of healthcare professionals. Typically, an oncological care pathway is both multidisciplinary and often cross-enterprise, including participants from different specialisms and different hospitals. In order to be able to work together and study the different patient cases, the participating specialists, radiologists, pathologists, nurses, and paramedics must have access to the relevant medical information. They also need an overview of the current status of the process to see whether the required information is available. We will talk about the new TBR process in detail. It is divided into 15 steps, described next.

Request TBR

The TBR requestor, after deciding to present the case in a tumor board for review, will create a new team in Microsoft Teams. Figure 5-8 shows how easy it is to create a new team for a specific tumor board review with three simple clicks. The TBR requestor should give an appropriate name for the TBR team, provide a description, and click "Next." The privacy option should be "Private - Only team owners can add team members" so that other members who are not part of this TBR cannot access the information stored inside this team space. Figure 5-8 shows how to request a TBR.

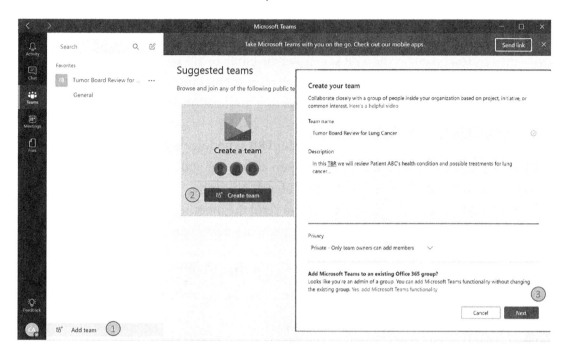

Figure 5-8. *MS Teams, request TBR*

After creating a team, the requestor can add TBR members if known at that point in time, else they can add a scheduler so that the TBR scheduler can start identifying and adding team members. The requestor then can start uploading all the relevant materials, such as documents, images, or reports, to the Files tab inside the newly created team (Figure 5-9).

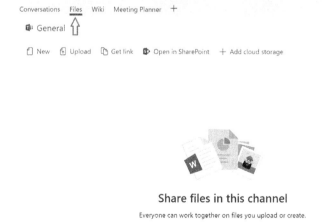

Figure 5-9. *MS Teams, Files tab*

Schedule TBR

Once the request is sent to the TBR scheduler via email or via Teams notification, the TBR scheduler can start the process of adding relevant members and documents, check everyone's schedule, and send the meeting notification to all members via team calendar.

The important part to note here is that the TBR scheduler is not going anywhere else, staying in the same MS Teams space to do all his/her activities mentioned. This increases the productivity of the TBR scheduler significantly.

Figure 5-10 shows how the scheduler can send the meeting notification to the added team members in Teams and how the other team members can view it.

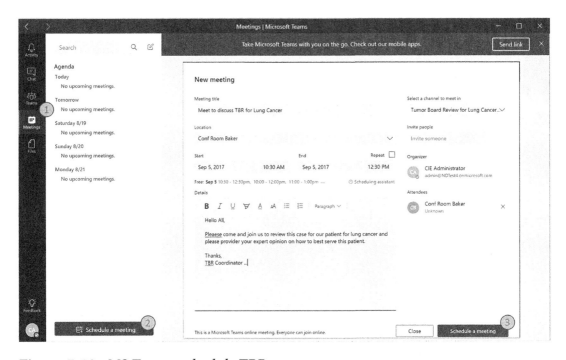

Figure 5-10. *MS Teams, schedule TBR*

This screen shows how the TBR scheduler can schedule a meeting with all team members in three simple clicks. Table 5-3 provides the description of each field and why selecting the right information is important.

Table 5-3. *Fields to Consider While Scheduling a Tumor Board Review*

Field Name	Description	Notes
Meeting Title	Title of the meeting, which members will see when they receive the invitation	
Location	This can be the conference room available for the duration of the meeting	This information will come from Azure AD and all the rooms' identities are synced from on-premises AD to Azure AD
Start Date	Meeting start date and time	
End Date	Meeting end date and time	
Repeat	If this meeting needs to be repeated in the future then this can be checked	
Details	Body text of the invitation that will be sent to all the members	
Select a channel to meet in	This is the team space for which scheduler is creating a meeting.	Important: Once scheduler selects the right team space, the meeting invitation will be sent to everyone in that team. No need to select individual members and send separate meeting requests.
Invite People	Invite people who are not part of the original team, such as a specialist who will be part of just this meeting but will not contribute throughout the lifecycle of the TBR process	
Organizer	Person who is scheduling the meeting, TBR scheduler	
Attendees	This field will include conference rooms and all the invited people	

Once the meeting is scheduled, the scheduler can go back and make appropriate changes (Figure 5-11).

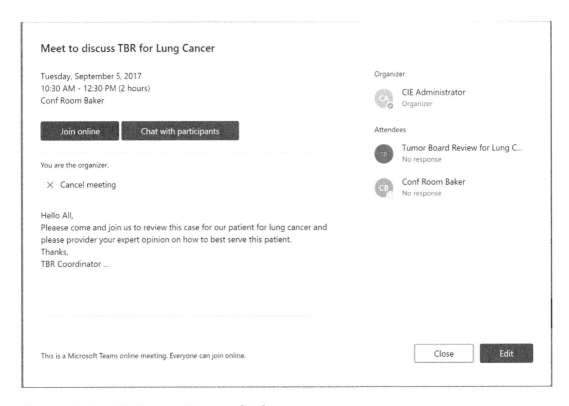

Figure 5-11. *MS Teams, View and Edit screen*

Prepare TBR

Once the meeting is scheduled and the invitation is sent, all of the participants can start collaborating with each other from the same Teams space. Figure 5-12 shows how the meeting will show up in the MS Teams interface for all the team members.

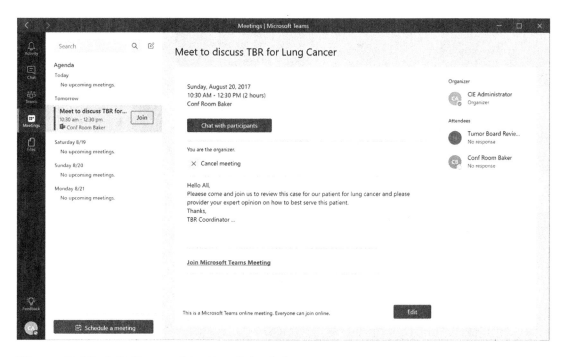

Figure 5-12. *MS Teams, Meeting Schedule screen*

Members can join this meeting by clicking on the "Join" button, which will start the voice/audio call with all the participants. Members can also instant message other members and start discussing the case. It is important to note here that all the conversations (instant messages) are stored within the same MS Teams space. MS Teams truly provides one single place for all conversations, documents, meetings, and conferences.

TBR Meeting

On the meeting day and time, all the participants can join the meeting from anywhere using any device, as long as they have access to the Teams space. Joining the meeting is as easy as clicking on the "Join" button. Figure 5-13 shows the screen participants will see upon joining the meeting.

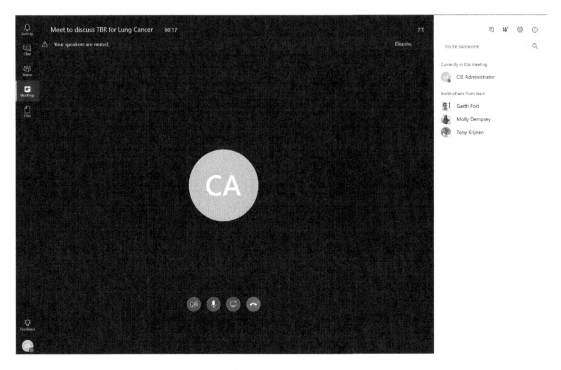

Figure 5-13. *MS Teams, meeting in action*

This is a very familiar interface for those who are familiar with the Skype application. Members can start the video call by unchecking the video icon ( ) shown in the preceding screen. Participants can also share their screen by clicking on the screen share icon ( ), shown above the screen. Typically, those who are leading the meeting will share their screen to take input from other participants. Meeting attendees can start taking notes using OneNote right from the MS Teams space. Figure 5-14 shows how OneNote can be used to take notes in real time. Meeting attendees can start collaborating on those notes during the meeting itself. There is no need to send the notes back to the attendees after the conference, which saves time and helps return the findings sooner to the TBR requestor.

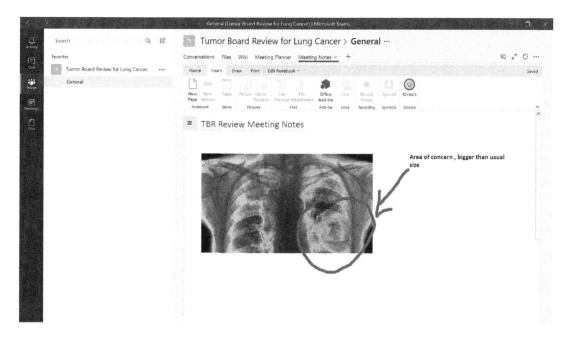

Figure 5-14. *MS Teams, OneNote tool*

OneNote helps with taking notes, copying images, and annotating on the images in real time. This helps specialists drill down on the area of concern and quickly come to a conclusion on a treatment approach. Teams can help search for similar cases and content from within the same interface. During a review board, there are many times when it is necessary to look for similar cases and the outcomes of those cases. Teams helps with this instant search for people, messages, and files from the same interface so that board members don't have to leave the Teams interface.

Finalize TBR

After everyone reviews and agrees on a recommended treatment, final notes can be saved and shared with the TBR requestor. The TBR requestor can check all the updated notes, conversations, documents, and treatment recommendations and make appropriate adjustments to the patient's treatment. The TBR scheduler can also send a survey using SurveyMonkey by adding a new tab to the same Teams space. Figure 5-15 shows how to add SurveyMonkey as a new tab to the same Teams meeting space.

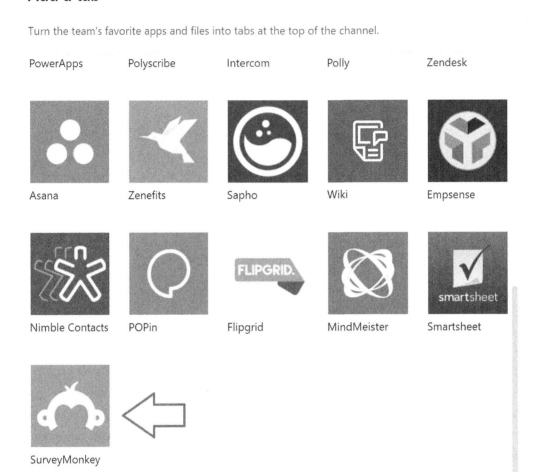

Add a tab   ×

Turn the team's favorite apps and files into tabs at the top of the channel.

PowerApps   Polyscribe   Intercom   Polly   Zendesk

Asana   Zenefits   Sapho   Wiki   Empsense

Nimble Contacts   POPin   Flipgrid   MindMeister   Smartsheet

SurveyMonkey

Add Excel spreadsheet tabs you can easily get to.

Figure 5-15. *MS Teams, add a survey tab*

As shown in the figure, Teams can integrate into the Office 365 Planner app as well. Planner can help with creating tasks for each of the participants as well as for patients. Planner can add tasks for nurses for required patient visits, assign tasks to patients for doctor's appointment, create tasks for physicians for patient visits, assign tasks to clinicians for laboratory tests in the future, send alerts and notifications, and keep track of the progress of overall treatment. This new process helps the TBR process shrink from days and weeks to a few hours, with higher accuracy and fewer communication gaps.

Conclusion

Tumor boards are not new, but there are still inefficiencies that can be tackled via tools like MS Teams, as explained in this chapter. With more tumor boards, more cancer patients would be able to get the opinion of all disciplines. With technology innovations, tumor boards can be more accessible to a larger community of physicians, and more patients can benefit from them. With the help of technology, physicians can make better educated judgments about the management of patients' care. TBRs also help with increasing cooperation and trust between physicians, as well as between allied health professionals. A TBR can be the most valuable educational tool available for the hospital staff and the cornerstone of a successful community cancer program.

In the future, next-generation technologies like augmented reality, artificial intelligence (AI), robotics, and the Internet of Things (IOT) can contribute to TBRs, making them even more realistic. Imagine TBR members are reviewing a patient's medical images using HoloLenses while in various facilities, all for a patient who is located in a remote location or even internationally. NASA rover scientists are using HoloLenses to walk around and explore Mars right from their offices. Surgical teams can use them to simulate a complex surgery during a TBR to improve the outcome of the treatment. TBR members can record the upcoming procedure and give patients a better understanding of what that upcoming procedure looks like. Artificial intelligence (AI) can match all the images from the past TBR and provide proactive suggestions on treatment for a given case during the TBR process. AI can help improve the diagnosis of diseases by looking at 30 years' worth of past similar cases in just a few minutes. AI can give extra ammunition to clinicians to battle a disease outbreak and can help find the cure faster. Robots have already started performing operations with the help of doctors. Robots can add precision to the procedure and improve the surgery results. Most of the new medical and clinical devices come with sensors that can automatically report many things, like the new beds in patient rooms. Most new patient beds have sensors that can tell if the patient is in the bed or not, the temperature of the room, and more. A TBR can be a good platform on which to test these future innovations and help improve medical outcomes. Hence, leveraging TBRs more often is advisable for any clinical trial.

CHAPTER 6

Overcome Scheduling Challenges

Nurse scheduling is about finding an optimal way to assign nurses to shifts and maintain the correct nurse-to-patient ratio at any given point in time at the hospital or facility. The nurse scheduling problem has been studied since at least 1969 and is a very complex problem that can be solved via algorithms. This chapter, however, will focus on solving this problem by putting the scheduling decisions in the hands of nurses and will not focus on solving it via any computer algorithms. Staffing and scheduling is not only a tiresome process but also requires nurse managers to have the right tools to predict the demand for nurses for any given shift hour. The primary responsibility of any nurse manager and chief nursing officer is to allocate the resources needed to deliver high-quality care at the right time to the right patient. Patients have different needs at various stages of their hospital stay. Maintaining a staffing ratio is a good starting point for any nurse manager but is not enough to provide high-value care to all admitted patients. Patients may range from needing minimal care on the day of their discharge to needing a dedicated nurse around the clock after a complication puts them in the ICU. The nurse manager needs new tools for creating staffing models and doing nurse scheduling and should have a way to pass on the responsibility to nurses for their own schedules. Nurse scheduling and ensuring each shift is staffed appropriately is one of the main reasons for job dissatisfaction among nurse managers. No matter how carefully the nurse manager defines the schedule criteria, there may always be holes in the schedule as it is dependent on a human element.

Nurse shortages, an aging nurse population, restrictive union contracts, and mandated staff-to-patient ratios are some of the big challenges every healthcare provider faces. Nurse managers must call nurses and request daily that they take on more shifts. Due to the long-term staff shortage, nurse managers must leverage external agencies to fill the gaps, which is usually very expensive and often creates friction with permanent

© Nidhish Dhru 2018
N. Dhru, *Office 365 for Healthcare Professionals*, https://doi.org/10.1007/978-1-4842-3549-2_6

staff due to the higher wages paid to agency nurses. To fill open shifts, organizations can offer incentives or bonuses to fulltime staff, but that often causes greater fatigue. Dissatisfied nurses often perform poorly or look elsewhere for other options, and that increases the turnover rates. Nurses commonly lack control over their own scheduling and staffing. Recruiting and retaining nurses gets even more difficult if their preferences are overlooked. Nurses need flexibility on where and when they work, selective overtime, and the ability to float between units. On top of nurses' preferences, regulatory and union requirements make scheduling and staffing even more complicated. Organizations have to be sensitive to regulatory requirements such as number of hours worked, overtime, time off, certifications, staffing ratios, and credentials being in accordance with standards set by the Joint Commission on Accreditation of Healthcare Organizations (JCAHO).

The Nurse Staffing and Inpatient Hospital Mortality study reported that hospitals with higher registered nurse staffing had lower rates of urinary tract infection, pneumonia, shock, and upper gastrointestinal bleeding, as well as shorter hospitalizations compared to hospitals with low numbers of registered nurses. Nurse staffing and scheduling is paramount for better patient outcomes and higher nurse satisfaction.[1]

Staffing Challenge

On average a nurse manager starts scheduling shifts four to eight weeks in advance considering the size of the organization. Even after planning well in advance, there are variables that impact that planning, such as time off requests, emergency leave, sick calls, and other personal reasons. Nurse managers are always juggling between budget constraints and hiring agency staff for temporary needs to fill the shifts. Available nurses are forced to keep up a blistering pace to take care of patients in timely manner. This, over time, results into burnt-out nurses, dissatisfied patients, and medical errors. Self-scheduling is one of the main asks from staff nurses as they want to take control of where and when they work. Nurse scheduling in practice often overlooks staff preferences, which results into lower staff satisfaction, higher attrition, and difficulties in hiring. We can divide these constraints into two categories: hard constraints and soft constraints.

[1] Jack Needleman, Ph.D., Peter Buerhaus, Ph.D., R.N., V. Shane Pankratz, Ph.D., Cynthia L. Leibson, Ph.D., Susanna R. Stevens, M.S., and Marcelline Harris, Ph.D., R.N., *New England Journal of Medicine*, 2011(364):1037–1045, March 17, 2011, DOI: 10.1056/NEJMsa1001025

Hard constraints are the constraints that, if failed, invalidate the entire schedule. Hard constraints typically include a specification of shifts (e.g., morning, afternoon, and night), that each nurse should work no more than one shift per day, and that all patients should have nursing coverage. Having differences in qualifications between nurses also creates hard constraints by allowing only certified nurses to provide care to a specific category of patients. A nurse does not do a late-night shift followed by a day shift the next day.

Soft constraints are the constraints that are desirable, but not meeting them does not make the schedule invalid. Soft constraints may include the minimum and maximum number of shifts assigned to a given nurse in each week, hours worked per week, days worked consecutively, and consecutive days off, as well as the shift preferences of individual nurses, or a nurse may go on vacation and will not work shifts during this time.

Solution Approach

Many organizations are turning to technology to help them resolve such staffing challenges. Some organizations have invested in giving scheduling control to the nurses, therefore decreasing nurse managers' workloads and increasing flexibility for nurses, which raises their level of satisfaction. Such tools can help nurses willingly give more time to their organization and help reduce staffing challenges. A benefit of giving the power of scheduling and rescheduling to nurses is that it enables nurses to assign themselves to shifts and units where their skills are most utilized. Nurse managers can oversee the scheduling and can also provide their input where appropriate.

Healthcare providers usually have many facilities and geographically distributed environments. The traditional approach of deploying a centralized solution will no longer work in an environment that seeks flexibility, simplicity, and accessibility. Many providers are turning to a cloud-based system (accessed via the internet), which gives them simplicity in terms of deployment and maintenance, flexibility in terms of adding/removing resources to and from that system, and accessibility in terms of securely accessing the system from anywhere using any device at any time. In the past, each hospital had to install its own tools locally for nurse scheduling, which never talked to other hospitals, operating solo. For nurses who provided care in multiple facilities, their nurse managers had to go through a manual process to make sure their schedule aligned between facilities. Shift bidding or shift posting across sites can greatly help internal staff resources. Flexibility in scheduling increases the pool of available staff to cover those shifts and helps reduce overtime as well as the need for external short-term staff. All of these factors influence staff satisfaction and, ultimately, turnover and retention rates. Nurse managers no longer must spend time on the phone begging, cajoling, and pleading.

The following section will describe one such tool, StaffHub, which is available as part of the Office 365 product suite. Licensing of this tool is not covered in this chapter, as licensing terms and conditions vary customer by customer, and arrangements must be made between Microsoft and the customer.

StaffHub

Microsoft StaffHub is designed as a scheduling agent to help nurses and nurse managers schedule shifts more efficiently even as their own jobs require them to be on their feet or on the go. StaffHub helps with creating and managing work shifts, sharing files, and communicating important information with team members. It's available to Office 365 for Business subscribers and comes with a web app for managers and mobile app for employees. The mobile app supports both iOS and Android. Nurse managers can use the StaffHub web app to create schedules, manage requests for shift swaps or time off, and share information with the team. Nurses can use the mobile app to view their shifts, submit shift and time-off requests, and communicate with the team.

StaffHub helps with overcoming the unique challenges nurses face every day in the clinical environment. Because of work pressure, nurses often feel disconnected from the team and company on the latest news and improvements. Nurses are often behind on the latest trainings, practices, procedures, processes, and tools due to the lack of time in a workday. Because of their busy schedules, nurses also receive information slower, do not know much about additional resources available to them, and cannot follow the latest updates on policies and governance standards. StaffHub helps in all these situations via schedule and task management, connecting a wide range of nurses via communications and community, and providing the latest information on training and onboarding activities, while keeping all this information secured via identity and access management.

Accessing StaffHub

To access the StaffHub portal, follow these steps:

1. Go to `https://staffhub.ms`.

2. Log in with your work credentials.

3. You should see the screen in Figure 6-1 upon successful login.

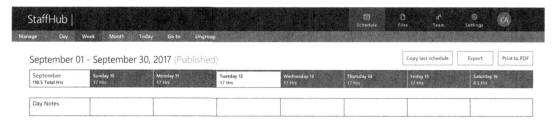

Figure 6-1. *Nurse Manager view, landing page*

Easily Create and Manage Schedules

Standard practice at most hospitals is to print out the schedules and stick them on bulletin boards either in breakrooms or in the lobby. Nurse managers can use color coding to designate specific shift types (such as opening, closing, and swing shifts) or responsibilities. Nurse managers can save time each week by clicking the convenient "Copy Last Schedule" button to quickly create next week's schedule from this week's.

Nurse managers can easily create and manage schedules for nurses, mark time off, move or copy shifts, and track vacation, sick leave, and other off-work requests as shown in Figure 6-2. Nurse managers can go to a specific week to assign shifts and schedule their time. They can create groups for creating different shifts. These shifts will be stored for future use. As shown in the figure, nurse managers can create different groups for morning and night shifts.

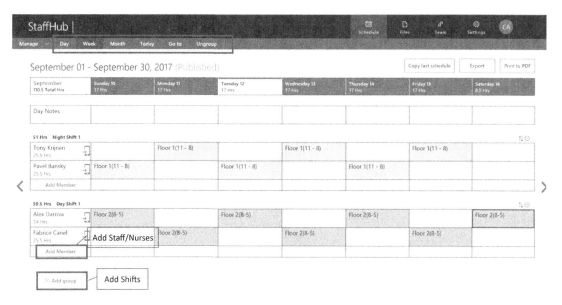

Figure 6-2. *Nurse Manager view, create and manage shedules*

After creating a schedule, the nurse manager can start adding members/nurses for that shift. The nurse manager can assign breaks, duties, and time off to members while assigning them to a shift. They can also assign different colors to shifts to visually identify morning and night shifts. Figure 6-3 shows how a nurse manager can create or manage shifts.

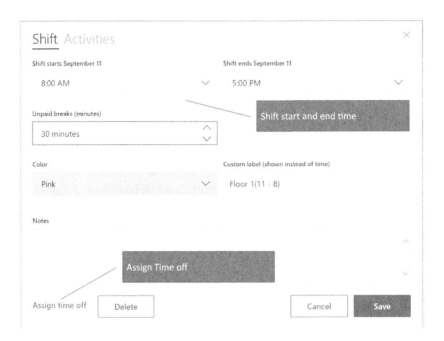

Figure 6-3. *Nurse Manager, create and manage shifts*

The nurse manager can start assigning activities for each shift of any length, classify those activities as paid or unpaid, and assign codes and colors to easily identify activities across hundreds of activities between main shifts. Figure 6-4 shows how a nurse manager can assign activities for each shift.

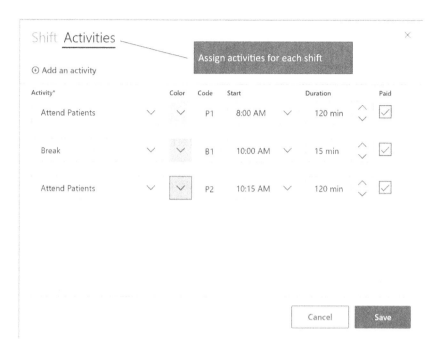

Figure 6-4. *Nurse Manager, assign tasks/activities to each shift*

StaffHub simplifies the process of handling schedule changes. After the nurse manager publishes the schedule, any changes that are made to it are immediately available to scheduled workers. Staff members can propose shift swaps among themselves and request time off directly from their mobile devices. Nurse managers always have the final say. They can approve or deny the request directly in StaffHub. Once a request is approved, StaffHub automatically updates the schedule. The nurse manager can create open shifts with a different color and note. Staff members as well as physicians can view the open shifts and request the assignment for that shift via the Conversation tab in their mobile app. Conversations carried out via the StaffHub app reduce the number of calls the nurse manager has to make for shift confirmations or shift swaps; all communication can be managed from one single app, which every stakeholder can view. Nurse managers can create schedules for different locations in the same schedule calendar to make sure there is no double-booking or over-booking of staff. Staff can also schedule their shifts right from the app to save time and reduce headaches for both nurses and schedulers. The biggest advantage of using a system like StaffHub is that it gives time back to nurse managers for value-add activities instead of bogging them down in the day-to-day tactics of scheduling, canceling, calling, trading shifts, and so forth. Some organizations do not allow their employees to use personal phones or other devices to access organization data via applications. Chapter 2 explains how to restrict access to Office 365 applications such as StaffHub from home; see the "Conditional Access" section.

Add or Remove Staff

After creating a schedule, the nurse manager can start assigning staff to that schedule. StaffHub allows managers to leverage Office 365 accounts as StaffHub is integrated with Office 365. Office 365 accounts (staff/physicians/nurse managers) can have access to collaboration resources, communication channels, files sharing, and more. StaffHub provisions an Office 365 group for every team that a nurse manager creates, allowing them to easily set up a collection of resources for staff. Managers don't have to worry about manually assigning permissions to all those resources, as adding members to the group automatically gives them the permissions they need to access the tools the group provides.

To enable the self-provisioning of accounts, log in to `https://staffhub.office.com/admin` using the administrator work account. Figure 6-5 shows how to set up the self-provisioning of accounts.

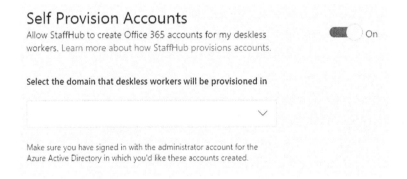

Figure 6-5. *Enable Self Provision Accounts from Staffhub admin portal*

After allowing StaffHub to self-provision accounts, nurse managers can start adding staff to the schedule. Adding new workers to your team, assigning shifts to them, and provisioning them with the resources they need to do their jobs can be a time-consuming task for a manager. Adding a new worker to the team is as easy as clicking "Add Team Member" on the Team tab, entering the new worker's phone number, and clicking "Add." After adding new team members, the manager can assign shifts to them and send each of them an invitation to StaffHub. Staff members can easily accept the invitation, download the mobile app, and access the resources they need to do their jobs—all from their mobile devices via StaffHub. Figure 6-6 shows how to add team members to existing teams.

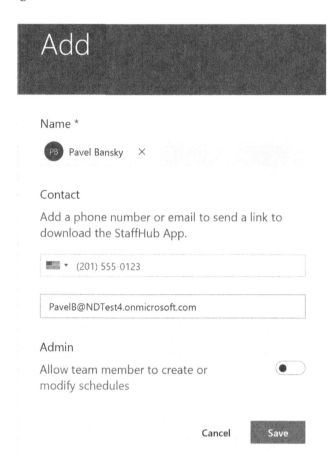

Figure 6-6. *Add team members to existing teams*

Managers can also remove staff members from the team easily. From the Team tab, select the team member you want to delete and click on the trash icon (Figure 6-7).

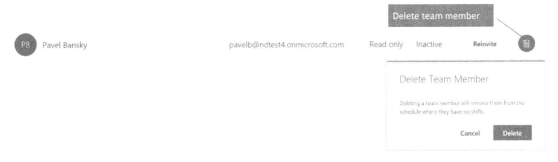

Figure 6-7. *Delete team member from existing team*

Removing a team member from the team will remove the team member from all future schedules where he or she has not been assigned to a shift. If the worker has been assigned to shifts, those shift cells in the schedule appear with a gray diagonal bar through them to show that the worker assigned to those shifts has been removed. That way, you can easily reassign the worker's shifts without disrupting the rest of the schedule.

Create Groups for Easier Scheduling

Nurse managers can create group schedules to simplify the process of scheduling staff across multiple departments or functions. Staff members can be part of more than one group if the nurse works for more than one department. Groups help in organizing team members by role or department in the schedule. Figure 6-8 shows where to add groups and members.

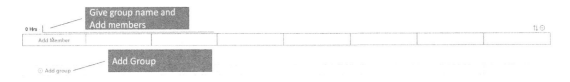

Figure 6-8. *Create groups*

Export or Print Schedules

Nurse managers can export the StaffHub schedule as an Excel file or print it out as a PDF for compliance and analysis perspective. Nurse managers can calculate overtime and extra pay for nurses, and the organization can calculate extra pay for physicians working on public holidays or odd hours. Nurse managers can also figure out the overall budget required to sustain the available staff or to decide to either increase or decrease the staff. The exported report can show the daily total hours burn rate per staff member or per shift. Reports can also show total time off, sick leave, and so forth if managed well in StaffHub. Figure 6-9 shows how to export the report to Excel or print it as a PDF.

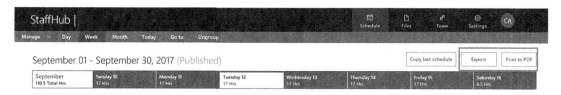

Figure 6-9. *Export or print as PDF*

This exported report can also be used to generate timesheet data for payroll. Both the report and the portal show actual time worked by nurses for the entire month to determine any payroll adjustments. The nurse manager or nurse can add notes explaining deviations or overtime for the payroll team so they can calculate extra pay or deduct the pay. Nurse managers can print the schedule and stick it to a common-area board for nurses to quickly check their shift and notes.

Access Scheduling Information from Any Device

Once a nurse manager adds a nurse to a shift, that nurse will get an email or text invitation. The nurse will have to follow the process listed in the email to install the StaffHub application on their mobile device. Once it is installed, the nurse can open the app and sign in with his or her Office 365 work account. He or she can view and manage their current and upcoming shifts on the My Shifts tab. Nurses can view their schedules in any web browser by signing in to StaffHub, but cannot manage their schedules unless given permission to do so. The StaffHub app will allow nurses to view their schedules from anywhere using any device at any time with high-level security. Nurses and physicians will have access to their schedules 24/7 from home or hospital, from desktop or mobile devices. The nurse manager controls who will be allowed access and which nurse/physician self-service features will be enabled for managing schedules. Figure 6-10 shows the mobile view of the StaffHub app.

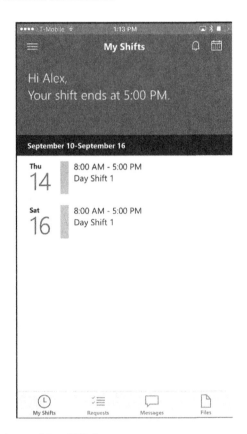

Figure 6-10. *Mobile view of StaffHub app*

Swap Shifts with Another Nurse or Physician

Personal emergencies happen, and staff must be able to change their work schedules to take care of such instances. The nurse manager must be flexible and accommodate shift changes to not adversely impact staff morale. Putting control in the hands of staff to decide whom they want to switch shifts with, and having other staff members accept the shift changes, is critical for running the day-to-day operations smoothly. StaffHub helps by providing an easy-to-use shift-swapping interface with notifications that get sent to the manager as well as to the person to whom the new shift is assigned. The nurse manager and the staff both can view the available staff during that shift via the schedule interface. StaffHub provides a notification in the app as well as on their devices. Figure 6-11 shows how to switch shifts.

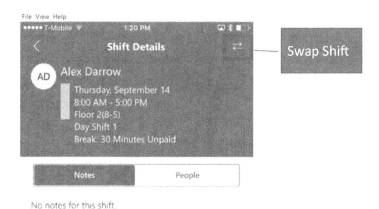

Figure 6-11. *Swap shift*

Staff/Nurse (Alex, in this case) can click on the Swap Shift icon to swap the shift with another staff member. Alex can find out who else is available to swap the shift with using the same interface shown in Figure 6-12.

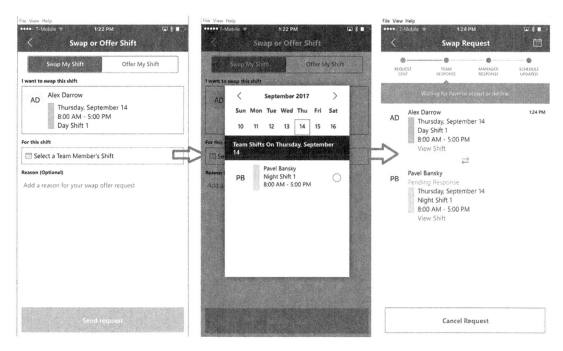

Figure 6-12. *Swap shift with Pavel Bansky*

Alex can see who is available on his team to swap the shift with. Alex can select one of the team members (Pavel, in this case) and send a request to Pavel to swap the shift. Pavel will receive the notification on his mobile device about a swap-shift request from Alex. Pavel can go to his StaffHub app from his mobile device to either approve or reject the request, as shown in Figure 6-13.

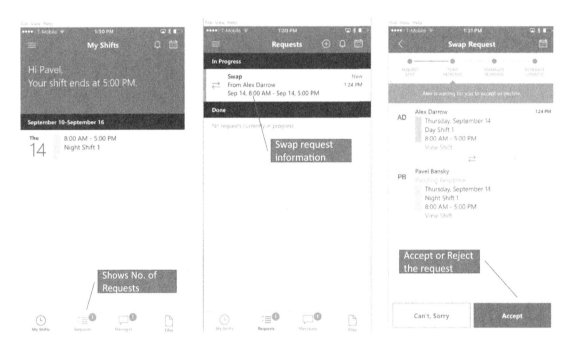

Figure 6-13. *Pavel Bansky can accept or reject the request*

Once Pavel accepts the request, the nurse manager will get notified about the shift swap. The manager can decide to accept or reject the request. Once the manager approves it, Alex can finally see his shift is swapped with his teammate, as shown in Figures 6-14 and 6-15.

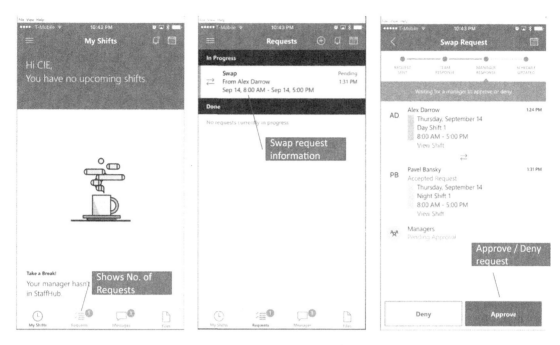

Figure 6-14. *Nurse Manager view to approve or deny the request*

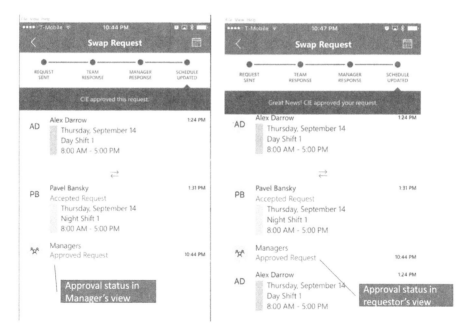

Figure 6-15. *Nurse Manager and Nurse views after reqeust is approved*

Once the request is approved, all the parties will be notified, and the shift changes are made.

Request Time Off

Staff can request paid or unpaid time off for an upcoming vacation, family leave, or other reason via the same StaffHub app. The approval workflow will start once the request is made for time off. The nurse can log in to the StaffHub application with his or her work account ID. Once logged in, the nurse can select the Requests icon at the bottom of the screen and request time off, as shown in Figure 6-16.

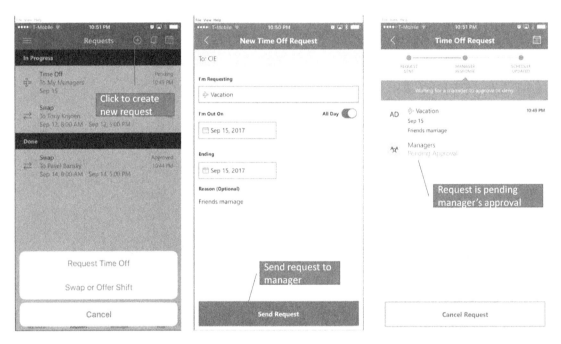

Figure 6-16. *Nurse requesting time off*

The nurse manager will get a notification on the schedule portal for a time-off request, as shown in Figure 6-17.

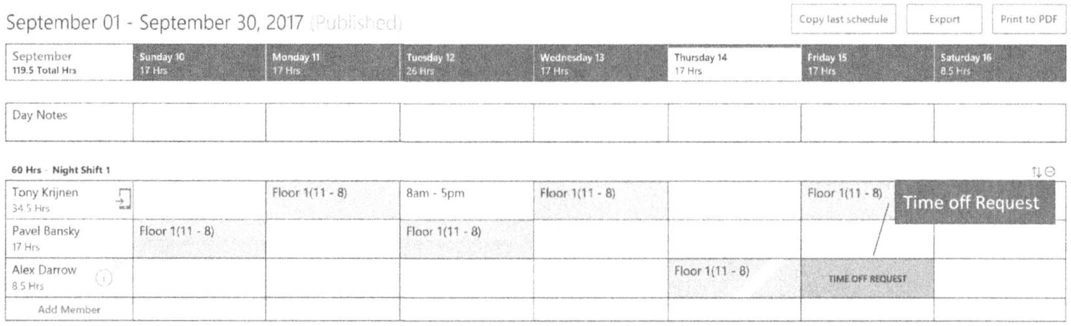

Figure 6-17. *Nurse Manager view for time-off request*

The nurse manager, based on the availability of staff at that shift, will either approve or deny the request, as shown in Figure 6-18.

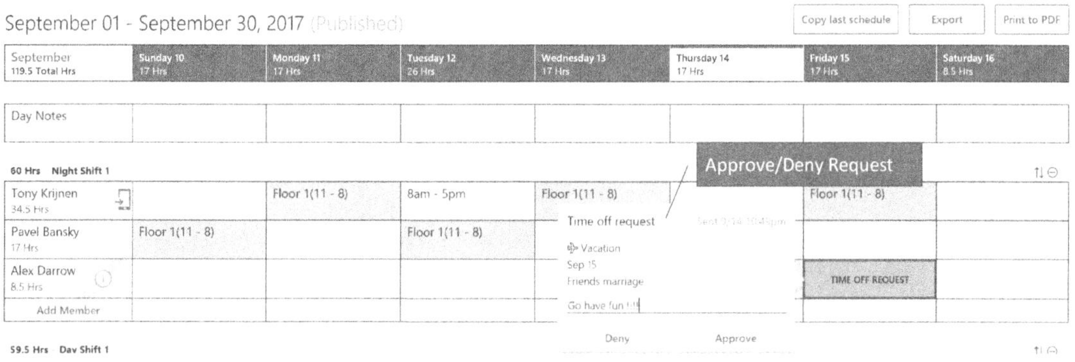

Figure 6-18. *Nurse Manager view for time-off request approval*

Once the approval is given, the nurse's schedule is marked as Vacation. Nurses can see the approval status and are automatically alerted when their request is approved or rejected via an iOS/Android in-app notification. The nurse manager, while exporting the schedule report, will be able to see all the time-off requests for a given staff member and can provide that information to the payroll department for appropriate action.

Training and Announcements

A busy schedule and constant work pressure keeps nurses very focused on patient care and better outcomes. Training is often neglected, as a result of which nurses are not always up to date on organizational changes, the latest procedures, and new governance policies. It can cause significant compliance violations as well as poor patient outcomes if nurses are not trained in a timely manner. Helping nurses take training from anywhere using any device securely can help them stay current with all the requirements. StaffHub offers a Files tab where the nurse manager can upload all the required training videos or documents, which nurses can access from their mobile devices via the StaffHub app, as shown in Figure 6-19.

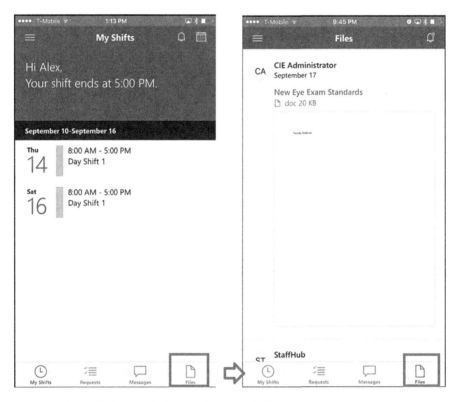

Figure 6-19. *Files tab for training videos and documents*

The nurse manager can communicate the training requirements or other important announcements via the Messages tab. Every time the nurse manager or other colleague sends a message to the shift team members, they all get a notification in their StaffHub app. The nurse can either respond to those messages right from the same interface or start a new conversation. There is no need to find out the phone numbers of the nurses to whom the message needs to be delivered or to text or call those nurses. The StaffHub app does all of that when someone posts a message in the Messages tab. This saves time for the nurse manager as he or she doesn't have to call each shift member individually; StaffHub simply broadcasts the message to all those who are assigned to the same shift, as shown in Figure 6-20.

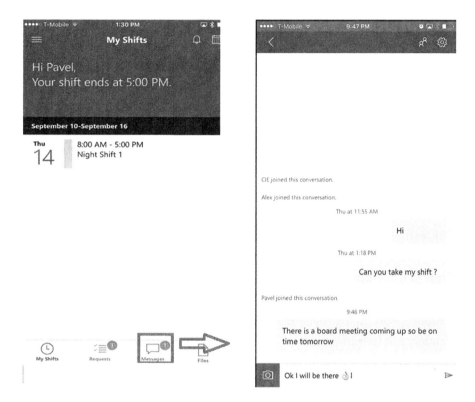

Figure 6-20. *Messages tab for announcements and chat*

Integration with Workforce Management Systems

Many providers use multiple systems and tools to help manage their workforce, such as applications like Kronos, a leading provider of workforce management and human capital management cloud solutions. Currently, StaffHub is not very well integrated with the Kronos system, but in the future it will be. This integration will enable managers to import individual and team schedule information from Kronos's Workforce Central platform directly into Microsoft StaffHub. This will help save time and money. StaffHub also supports the ability for nurse managers to define custom links for nurses to view in the mobile app, which can point to important resources or sites, such as HR systems for reporting time off or training sites for mandatory training, or even to custom applications built with tools such as Microsoft PowerApps.

Conclusion

Nurse staffing and scheduling is a complex problem every healthcare organization faces. Leveraging technology to help either solve or reduce the problem can help organizations save both time and money in the long term. There are many cloud-based solutions out there in the market, but they all act alone and provide no capability to integrate with existing productivity tools such as email, file sharing, communication, or Office documents. Organizations should adopt a strategy where they make the staffing and scheduling service part of the overall productivity platform for the easy integration and consistency of the information flow. More and more organizations are adopting a strategy where they give scheduling power to employees in order to reduce the burden on managers so that they can focus on more value-added services instead of mundane scheduling activities. As the emphasis on quality of care increases in healthcare organizations, every activity performed by managers has to be aligned with that emphasis on quality of care. If employees or managers are spending time that is ultimately not helping to improve quality of care, then organizations must take a real deep look at those activities and try to simplify them using the latest and greatest technology evolutions.

This chapter focused on providing a simplistic view of one such tool, StaffHub, which is part of the Office 365 suite. StaffHub not only is useful for those organizations that do not currently have any automated web-based tool for nurse scheduling, but can also help organizations that have invested in highly complex and expensive tools for nurse scheduling. StaffHub integrates easily with existing productivity tools such as email, file shares, communications, and Office documents, as it builds on top of the same platform as Office 365. Allowing users to access their schedules in real time via mobile devices at any time makes StaffHub even more acceptable in healthcare organizations, and especially to those who are constantly on the move. Providing simplicity when swapping shifts or requesting time off helps save time and money for healthcare organizations. StaffHub offers simplicity, ease of use, and universal access, which makes it a viable solution for the nurse-scheduling challenges faced by many healthcare organizations.

CHAPTER 7

Personal Health Record: External Sharing in a Secure Manner

As we know, sharing vital patient information in a timely manner can improve decision making at the point of care and help providers avoid readmissions and medication errors, improve diagnoses, and decrease duplicate testing. Electronic health-information exchange allows nurses, physicians, pharmacists, other healthcare providers, and patients to appropriately access and securely share a patient's vital medical information electronically to improve the speed, quality, safety, and cost of patient care. Most Americans' medical information is stored on paper despite the widespread availability of secure electronic data transfer. Patient data is in filing cabinets at various medical offices or in boxes and folders in patients' homes. Often, a patient carries their records from appointment to appointment, or information is shared between providers via mail, fax, or CDs. Patient and provider direct interaction is absolutely needed, but having electronic access to patients' health history is extremely beneficial for doctors and nurses for accurate diagnosis and speedy recovery. Electronic data transfer helps standardize patient data across multiple electronic health record (EHR) systems, thus improving the interoperability between multiple providers.

There are three ways patient data can be electronically exchanged between providers, as shown in Table 7-1.

© Nidhish Dhru 2018
N. Dhru, *Office 365 for Healthcare Professionals*, https://doi.org/10.1007/978-1-4842-3549-2_7

Table 7-1. *Patient Data Exchange Methods*

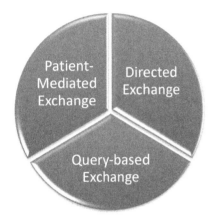

Directed Exchange

Directed exchange is when one provider sends information to another provider electronically easily and securely. An example of such a transaction could be laboratory orders and results, patient referrals, discharge summaries, and so on. The internet is the primary medium for this data transfer, and it is done in an encrypted format so that no third party can interfere in that transaction. Data transfer is usually between trusted parties, like two providers who send information back and forth via encrypted emails. This way of data transfer can enable coordinated care and benefits both providers and patients.

Such a directed data exchange could be a primary care provider directly sending electronic care summaries that include medications, problems, and lab results to a specialist when referring their patients. This information helps to inform the visit and prevents the duplication of tests, redundant collection of information from the patient, wasted visits, and medication errors. Directed exchange can also be used for sending immunization data to public-health organizations or to report quality measures to global organizations.

Query-based Exchange

Query-based exchange is when a physician is querying the data source of a patient's clinical record of any unplanned ad hoc care. Emergency room physicians can use query-based exchange to access patient information like medication history, past radiology images, known allergies to any medication, and so on, with the purpose of accurately prescribing medication so as to avoid adverse medication reactions or duplicative lab tests. When a pregnant patient goes to the hospital, query-based exchange can assist the physician in obtaining her pregnancy care record, allowing them to make safer decisions about the care of the patient and her unborn baby.

(continued)

Table 7-1. (*continued*)

	Patient-mediated Exchange
	In this type of data exchange, the patient is in control of his or her medical record. Patient-mediated data exchange provides patients with access to their health information, allowing them to manage their healthcare online in a similar fashion to how they might manage their finances through online banking. The patient can provide their health information to multiple providers, can identify or correct wrong or missing personal health information, can identify billing issues, and, most importantly, can choose to not share information with those whom they don't trust. However, HIPAA and other regulations have compelled providers to keep patient data in their safe deposit boxes, as the risk of data breaches can adversely impact patients and their health data.

There are three ways data can be transferred, as just shown. If the EHRs of two providers are integrated, then sharing information is relatively easy, as there is an inherent trust between the two systems. This chapter, however, focuses on scenarios where passing information between providers is done via papers, manually over the phone, or by CD. This is where SharePoint Online can play a big role. The following section will explain how a provider can secure the patient health information and share it externally with other providers via Office 365 and its services. Sharing content externally is very simple in SharePoint Online, as it provides logging and reporting capabilities to monitor the sharing of content. The following section will provide an approach for securely sharing content outside the organization by securing it first and then enabling the continuous monitoring of it from a compliance standpoint.

Protecting Patient Health Information (PHI)

SharePoint Online is a highly productive environment that is very intuitive for end users. SharePoint Online has built-in features like rights management, information protection via labeling, and data loss prevention, which make the environment highly secure and very productive. This chapter will showcase a few simple steps to secure patient information, share it externally, and continuously monitor it on an ongoing basis.

Disable External Sharing at Tenant Level

Providers can start using SharePoint Online and count on its being secure from day one. SharePoint environments can get big and messy very quickly due to its ease of use, so it is very important to keep the SharePoint Online environment in a good state from the get-go. Disabling external sharing from day one will help you ensure that no content is out of your hands. Figure 7-1 shows how to disable external sharing from the SharePoint Online Admin Center.

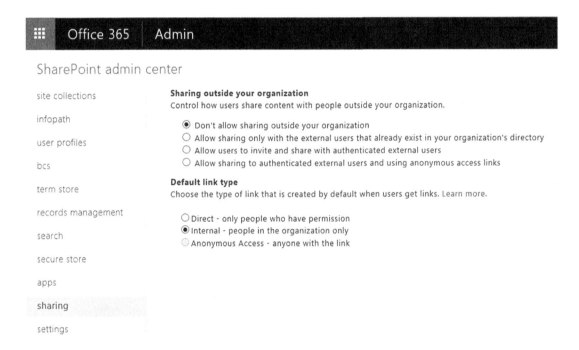

Figure 7-1. *Disable external sharing*

Enable Information Rights Management

Information rights management (IRM) limits the actions users can take on files after it's downloaded from SharePoint Online. IRM provides encryption for files so that no other user or program can open them unless given permission to do so. IRM protects files at the access level by controlling permissions at the user level and controlling actions such as printing or copying. IRM can be used on lists or libraries to limit the dissemination of sensitive content. For example, clinicians might create a document library to share information about patient health information with selected physicians and nurses; they can protect that library with IRM to prevent these individuals from sharing the content with other employees in the company or externally.

Clinicians can apply IRM to an entire list or library, rather than to individual files. This makes it easier to ensure a consistent level of protection for an entire set of documents or files. IRM can help providers enforce corporate policies that govern the use and dissemination of confidential or proprietary information.

IRM helps to protect restricted content in the following ways:

- Prevents an authorized viewer from copying, modifying, printing, faxing, or copying and pasting the content for unauthorized use

- Prevents an authorized viewer from copying the content by using the Print Screen feature in Microsoft Windows

- Prevents an unauthorized viewer from viewing the content if it is sent in an email after it is downloaded from the server

- Restricts access to content to a specified period, after which users must confirm their credentials and download the content again

- Helps to enforce corporate policies that govern the use and dissemination of content within your organization

IRM cannot protect restricted content from the following:

- Erasure, theft, capture, or transmission by malicious programs such as Trojan horses, keystroke loggers, and certain types of spyware

- Loss or corruption because of the actions of computer viruses

- Manual copying or retyping of content from the display on a screen

- Digital or film photography of content that is displayed on a screen

- Copying using third-party screen-capture programs

- Copying of content metadata (column values) through the use of third-party screen-capture programs or copy-and-paste action

Activate Rights Management

The following are the steps needed to activate rights management from the Office 365 Admin Center:

1. Sign in to the Office 365 Admin Center (`http://portal.office.com`).

2. Go to Admin portal.

3. Navigate to the Rights Management page or use the search functionality.

   - To navigate: Settings ➤ Services & add-ins ➤ Microsoft Azure Information Protection ➤ Manage Microsoft Azure Information Protection settings

   - To search: In the search box on the Home page, type *Information Protection*, and from the search results, click "Microsoft Azure Information Protection," and then choose "Manage Microsoft Azure Information Protection settings."

4. On the Rights Management page, click "Activate."

5. When prompted "Do you want to activate Rights Management?" click "Activate."

You should now see that rights management is activated, and the option to deactivate is available.

Rights Management Setup

After activating the rights management service, you must sign in to the SharePoint Admin Center to turn on information rights management (IRM).

1. Sign in to the Office 365 Admin Center (`http://portal.office.com`).

2. Choose Admin ➤ SharePoint. You're now in the SharePoint Admin Center.

3. Choose Settings.

4. On the Settings page, in the Information Rights Management (IRM) section, choose "Use the IRM service specified in your configuration," and then choose "Refresh IRM Settings."

SharePoint Online supports encryption of the following file types:

- PDF

- The 97–2003 file formats for the following Microsoft Office programs: Word, Excel, and PowerPoint

- The Office Open XML formats for the following Microsoft Office programs: Word, Excel, and PowerPoint

- The XML Paper Specification (XPS) format

Apply Rights Management to Document Library

The following are the steps to configure rights management at the document-library level:

1. Go to the list or library for which you want to configure IRM.

2. On the ribbon, click the Library tab, and then click the Library Settings icon as shown in Figure 7-2 (if you are working in a list, click the List tab and then click the List Settings icon).

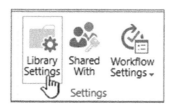

Figure 7-2. *Document library settings*

3. Under Permissions and Management, click "Information Rights Management." If this link does not appear, IRM might not be enabled for your site. Contact your server administrator to see if it is possible to enable IRM for your site. The "Information Rights Management" link does not appear for picture libraries.

4. On the Information Rights Management Settings page, select the "Restrict permission to documents in this library on download" checkbox to apply this restricted permission to documents that are downloaded from this list or library.

5. In the "Create a permission policy title" box, type a descriptive name for the policy that you can use later to differentiate this policy from other policies. For example, you can type *Company Confidential* if you are applying restricted permission to a list or library that will contain company documents that are confidential.

6. In the "Add a permission policy description" box, type a description that will appear to people who use this list or library that explains how they should handle the documents in this list or library. For example, you can type *Discuss the contents of this document only with other employees* if you want to restrict access to the information in these documents to internal employees.

7. To apply additional restrictions to the documents in this list or library, click "Show Options" and do any of the steps shown in Table 7-2).

Table 7-2. *Rights Management Configuration*

To do this:	Do this:
Allow people to print documents from this list or library	Select the "Allow viewers to print" checkbox.
Allow people with at least the View Items permission to run embedded code or macros on a document	Select the "Allow viewers to run script and screen reader to function on downloaded documents" checkbox. Note: If you select this option, users could run code to extract the contents of a document.
Require that people verify their credentials at specific intervals Select this option if you want to restrict access to content to a specified period. If you select this option, people's licenses to access the content will expire after the specified number of days, and people will be required to return to the server to verify their credentials and download a new copy.	Select the "Users must verify their credentials using this interval (days)" checkbox and then specify the number of days for which you want the document to be viewable.

(continued)

Table 7-2 (*continued*)

To do this:	Do this:
Prevent people from uploading documents that do not support IRM to this list or library. **If you select this option, people will not be able to upload any of the following file types:** **File types that do not have corresponding IRM protectors installed on all the front-end web servers** **File types that SharePoint Server 2010 cannot decrypt** **File types that are IRM protected in another program**	Select the "Do not allow users to upload documents that do not support IRM" checkbox.
Remove restricted permissions from this list or library on a specific date	Select the "Stop restricting access to the library" checkbox and then select the date that you want.
Control the interval at which credentials are cached for the program that is licensed to open the document	In the "Set group protection and credentials interval," enter the interval for caching credentials in number of days.
Allow group protection so that users can share with members of the same group	Select "Allow group protection" and enter the group's name for sharing.

Configure DLP Policies

To comply with business standards and industry regulations, organizations need to protect sensitive information and prevent its inadvertent disclosure. Examples of sensitive information that you might want to prevent from leaking outside your organization include financial data or personally identifiable information (PII), such as credit card numbers, social security numbers, or health records. With a data loss prevention (DLP) policy in the Office 365 Security & Compliance Center, you can identify, monitor, and automatically protect sensitive information across Office 365.

With a DLP policy, you can do the following:

- Identify sensitive information across many locations, such as Exchange Online, SharePoint Online, and OneDrive for Business.

  For example, you can identify any document containing a credit card number that's stored in any OneDrive for Business site, or you can monitor just the OneDrive sites of specific people.

- Prevent the accidental sharing of sensitive information.

  For example, you can identify any document or email containing a health record that's been shared with people outside your organization and then automatically block access to that document or block the email from being sent.

- Monitor and protect sensitive information in the desktop versions of Excel 2016, PowerPoint 2016, and Word 2016.

  Just like in Exchange Online, SharePoint Online, and OneDrive for Business, these Office 2016 desktop programs include the same capabilities to identify sensitive information and apply DLP policies. DLP provides continuous monitoring when people share content in these Office 2016 programs.

- Help users learn how to stay compliant without interrupting their workflow.

  You can educate your users about DLP policies and help them remain compliant without blocking their work. For example, if a user tries to share a document containing sensitive information, a DLP policy can both send them an email notification and show them a policy tip in the context of the document library that allows them to override the policy if they have a business justification. The same policy tips also appear in Outlook on the web, Outlook 2013 and later, Excel 2016, PowerPoint 2016, and Word 2016.

- View DLP reports showing content that matches your organization's DLP policies.

To assess how well your organization is complying with a DLP policy, you can see how many matches each policy and rule has had over time. If a DLP policy allows users to override a policy tip and report a false positive, you can also view what users have reported.

Create DLP Policy

Office 365 includes over 40 ready-to-use templates that can help you meet a wide range of common regulatory and business policy needs. For example, there are DLP policy templates for the following:

- Gramm-Leach-Bliley Act (GLBA)

- Payment Card Industry Data Security Standard (PCI-DSS)

- United States Personally Identifiable Information (US PII)

- United States Health Insurance Act (HIPAA)

    1.   Go to `https://protection.office.com`.

    2.   Sign in to Office 365 using your work or school account. You're now in the Office 365 Security & Compliance Center.

    3.   In the Security & Compliance Center ➤ Left navigation ➤ Data loss prevention ➤ Policy ➤ + Create a policy (as shown in Figure 7-3).

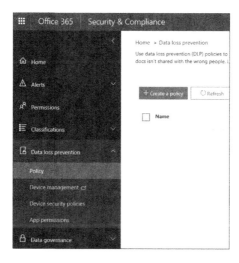

Figure 7-3. *Create a DLP policy*

4. Choose the DLP policy template that protects the types of
    sensitive information that you need and click "Next."

    In this example, you'll select Privacy ➤ US Health Insurance
    Act (HIPAA) Data because it already includes most of the types
    of sensitive information that you want to protect—you'll add a
    couple more later.

    When you select a template, you can read the description on the
    right to learn what types of sensitive information the template
    protects, as shown in Figure 7-4.

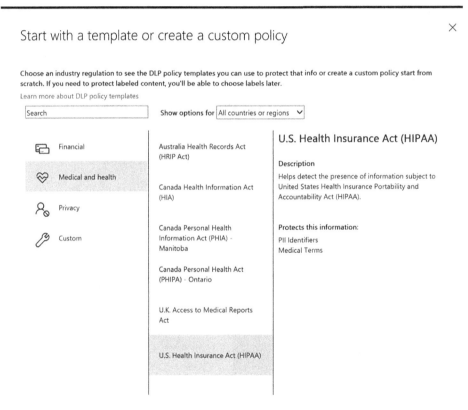

Figure 7-4. *Configure HIPAA DLP policy*

5. Name the policy and click "Next."

6. To choose the locations that you want the DLP policy to protect, do one of the following:

- Choose All locations in Office 365 ➤ Next.

- Choose Let me choose specific locations ➤ Next. For this example, choose this as shown in figure 7-5.

- To include or exclude an entire location, such as all Exchange emails or all OneDrive accounts, switch the status of that location on or off.

- To include only specific SharePoint sites or OneDrive for Business accounts, switch the Status to *on*, then click the links under "Include" to choose specific sites or accounts. When you apply a policy to a site, the rules configured in that policy are automatically applied to all sub-sites of that site, as shown in Figure 7-5.

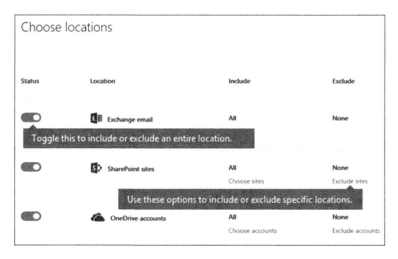

Figure 7-5. *Target SharePoint or OneDrive accounts*

In this example, to protect sensitive information stored in all OneDrive for Business accounts, turn off the Status for both Exchange emails and SharePoint sites and leave the Status on for OneDrive accounts.

7. Choose Use advanced settings ➤ Next.

8. A DLP policy template contains predefined rules with conditions and actions that detect and act upon specific types of sensitive information. You can edit, delete, or turn off any of the existing rules, or add new ones. When done, click "Next," as shown in Figure 7-6.

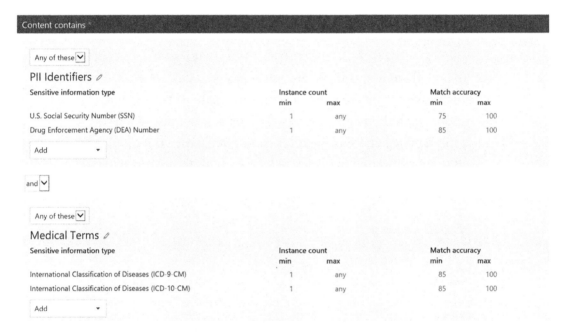

Figure 7-6. *DLP policy rules configuration*

To meet your organization's specific requirements, you may want to make the rules easier to trigger so that a single occurrence of sensitive information is enough to block access for external users.

9. Admins might not want DLP policies to block people from doing their work when they have a valid business justification or encounter a false positive, so you want the user notification to include options to override the blocking action.

In the "User notifications" section, you can see that email notifications and policy tips are turned on by default for this rule in the template.

In the "User overrides" section, you can see that overrides for a business justification are turned on, but overrides to report false positives are not. Choose "Override the rule automatically if they report it as a false positive," as shown in Figure 7-7.

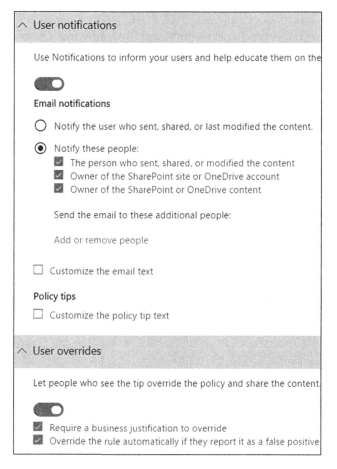

Figure 7-7. *DLP user notification*

10. At the top of the rule editor, change the name of this rule.

11. At the bottom of the rule editor select "Save."

12. Review the conditions and actions for this rule and click "Next."

On the right, notice the Status switch for the rule. If you turn off an entire policy, all rules contained in the policy are also turned off. However, here you can turn off a specific rule without turning off the entire policy. This can be useful when you need to investigate a rule that is generating many false positives.

13.   On the next page, read and understand the following, choose whether to turn on the rule or test it out first, then click "Next."

Before you create your DLP policies, you should consider rolling them out gradually to assess their impact and test their effectiveness before you fully enforce them. For example, you don't want a new DLP policy to unintentionally block access to thousands of documents that people require to get their work done.

View DLP Policies

Once the document is scanned for the DLP policy, if the document violates the policy, users will not be able to share the document with external users. As shown in Figure 7-8, a policy-violation message will appear with policy-tip details.

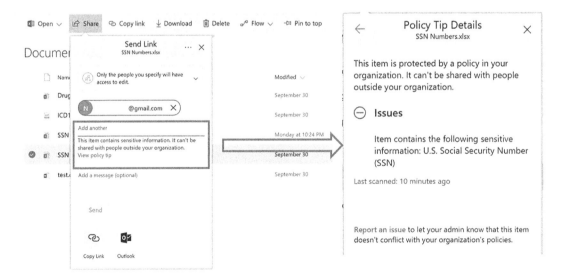

Figure 7-8. *DLP policy-violation icon*

DLP policies are synced to sites, and content is evaluated against them periodically and asynchronously, so there may be a short delay between the time you create the DLP policy and the time you begin to see policy tips. There may be a similar delay from when you resolve or override a policy tip to when the icon on the document on the site goes away.

Read more here: https://support.office.com/en-us/article/Send-email-notifications-and-show-policy-tips-for-DLP-policies-87496bc5-9601-4473-8021-cb05c71369c1?ui=en-US&rs=en-US&ad=US.

Develop "External Sharing Site Requests" List

Once external sharing is disabled and rights management is configured, it's time for users to make special requests if they absolutely must have external sharing sites. Admins can enable external sharing per site-collection level based on user requests. Create a list in the main/root site or a dedicated site where everyone has read and write access. Publish an "Add New Item" link to this list on the intranet homepage or communicate this via email to a broader audience. Just be sure to publish the link where every user can easily get to it and enter their request for an external sharing site.

Potential metadata for this list is shown in Table 7-3.

Table 7-3. *External Sharing List Metadata*

Column Name	Column Type	Description
Site Name	Text	This column should check the uniqueness of the site name.
Site Description	Text	This column should list the purpose of the site and potential users.
Site Administrator	People/Group	This column should list all the site-collection administrators for this site.
Keep it until	Date Time	This column should specify how long this site will be available.

Set Up Alerts

Once the list is created, set up an alert for the admin to tell them about anything newly added or changed. This should send an email notification to the admin for a new site request, and then the admin can take appropriate action, as shown in Figure 7-9.

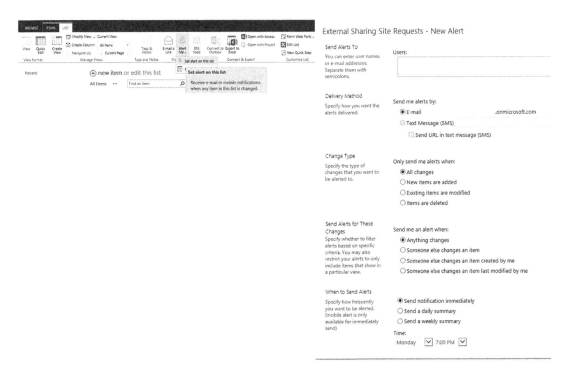

Figure 7-9. *Set up alerts on list/document library*

Workflow Setup

After setting up alerts for the admin, define a workflow for the approval. Most organizations have a governing body that decides who can share content outside and for what. This workflow can help with getting approval from those approvers before creating an external sharing site. A simple "Approval" workflow can help, but if your organization has more-specific needs then you can create complex workflows as well, as shown in Figure 7-10.

Workflow Details

Workflow

Select a workflow to add to this list. If a workflow is missing from the list, your site administrator may have to publish or activate it

Select a workflow template:

*Approval - SharePoint 2010
*Collect Feedback - SharePoint 2010
*Collect Signatures - SharePoint 2010
*Disposition Approval

Description:
Routes a document for approval. Approvers can approve or reject the document, reassign the approval task; or request changes to the document.

*Denotes a SharePoint 2010 template.

Name

Enter a name for this workflow. The name identifies this workflow.

Enter a unique name for this workflow:

Site Approvals

Task List

Select the name of the task list to use with this workflow, or create a new one.

Select a task list:

Workflow Tasks

Description:
This system library was created by the Publishing feature to store workflow tasks that are created in this site.

History List

Select the name of the history list to use with this workflow, or create a new one.

Select a history list:

Workflow History (new)

Description:
This workflow will use a new history list.

Start Options

Specify how this workflow can be started.

☑ Allow this workflow to be manually started by an authenticated user with Edit Item permis
☐ Require Manage Lists Permissions to start the workflow.

☐ Start this workflow to approve publishing a major version of an item.

☐ Creating a new item will start this workflow.

☐ Changing an item will start this workflow.

Approvers

Assign To | Order
| One at a time (serial) ☑

☐ Add a new stage
Enter the names of the people to whom the workflow will assign tasks, and choose the order in which those tasks are assigned. Separate them with semicolons. You ca also add stages to assign tasks to more people in different orders.

Expand Groups

☑ For each group entered, assign a task to every individual member and to each group that it contains.

Request

This message will be sent to the people assigned tasks.

Due Date for All Tasks

The date by which all tasks are due.

Duration Per Task

1

The amount of time until a task is due. Choose the units by using the Duration Units

Duration Units

Day(s)

Define the units of time used by the Duration Per Task.

CC

Notify these people when the workflow starts and ends without assigning tasks to them.

End on First Rejection ☑ Automatically reject the document if it is rejected by any participant.

End on Document Change ☑ Automatically reject the document if it is changed before the workflow is completed.

Enable Content Approval ☑ Update the approval status after the workflow is completed (use this workflow to control content approval).

Save | Cancel

Next

Figure 7-10. *Configure workflow*

Now you are ready to start accepting requests from users for external sharing sites. There are a few things you need to remember when you create a site.

By default, all SharePoint site collections have external sharing disabled, so you'll need to explicitly enable that as needed. You can easily automate this as part of your site collection provisioning tooling or manually by modifying the Sharing settings from the SharePoint Online Admin Portal as shown in Figure 7-11.

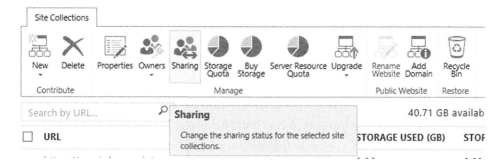

Figure 7-11. *Configure site collection–level sharing*

The actual popup for changing sharing settings is shown in Figure 7-12.

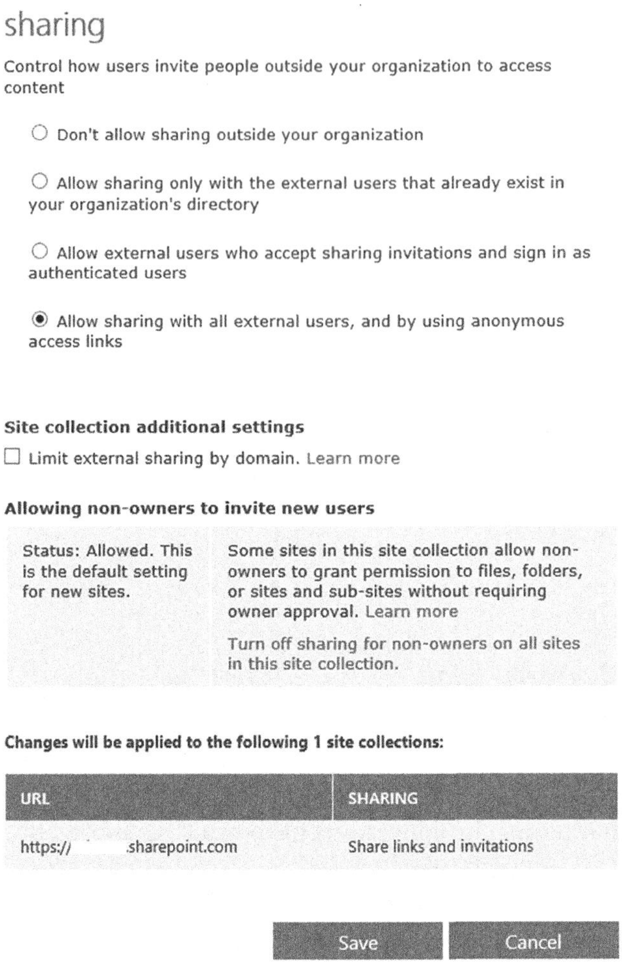

Figure 7-12. *Enable external sharing for site collection*

Configure Audit Settings

The audit feature of SharePoint Online lets admins track user actions on a site's content types, lists, libraries, list items, and library files within the site collections. Knowing who has done what with which information is critical for many business requirements, such as regulatory compliance and records management. Figure 7-13 shows how to configure audit settings.

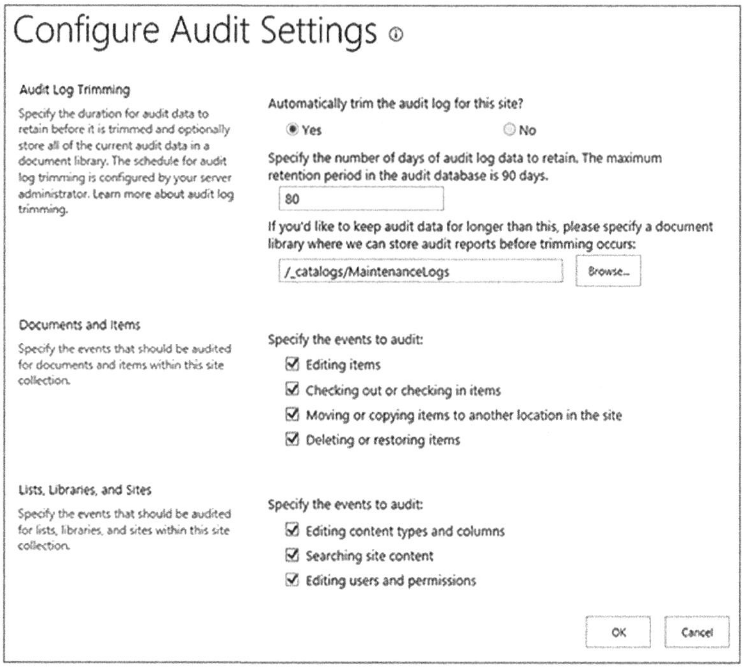

Configure Audit Settings ⓘ

Audit Log Trimming
Specify the duration for audit data to retain before it is trimmed and optionally store all of the current audit data in a document library. The schedule for audit log trimming is configured by your server administrator. Learn more about audit log trimming.

Automatically trim the audit log for this site?
  ⦿ Yes   ○ No

Specify the number of days of audit log data to retain. The maximum retention period in the audit database is 90 days.

  80

If you'd like to keep audit data for longer than this, please specify a document library where we can store audit reports before trimming occurs:

  /_catalogs/MaintenanceLogs   Browse...

Documents and Items
Specify the events that should be audited for documents and items within this site collection.

Specify the events to audit:
  ☑ Editing items
  ☑ Checking out or checking in items
  ☑ Moving or copying items to another location in the site
  ☑ Deleting or restoring items

Lists, Libraries, and Sites
Specify the events that should be audited for lists, libraries, and sites within this site collection.

Specify the events to audit:
  ☑ Editing content types and columns
  ☑ Searching site content
  ☑ Editing users and permissions

  [OK]   [Cancel]

Figure 7-13. *Configure audit settings*

You can manage the size of the audit log in the "Audit Log Trimming" section and specify which events to audit in the "Documents and Items" and "Lists, Libraries, and Sites" sections. You can also specify the maximum number of days that items will be retained. By default, all items are removed at the end of the month.

As a site-collection administrator, you can retrieve the history of actions taken by a user and also the history of actions taken during a date range. For example, you can determine which users edited a specific document and when they did this.

Configure Events to Audit

The following steps show how to configure events for audit for the SharePoint site:

1. Log in to a SharePoint site for which the admin needs to enable event auditing.

2. Select Settings ➤ Site settings.

3. If you are not at the root of your site collection, under "Site Collection Administration," select "Go to top level site settings."

Note The "Site Collection Administration" section will not be available if you do not have the necessary permissions.

4. On the Site Settings page, under "Site Collection Administration," select "Site collection audit settings" as shown in Figure 7-14.

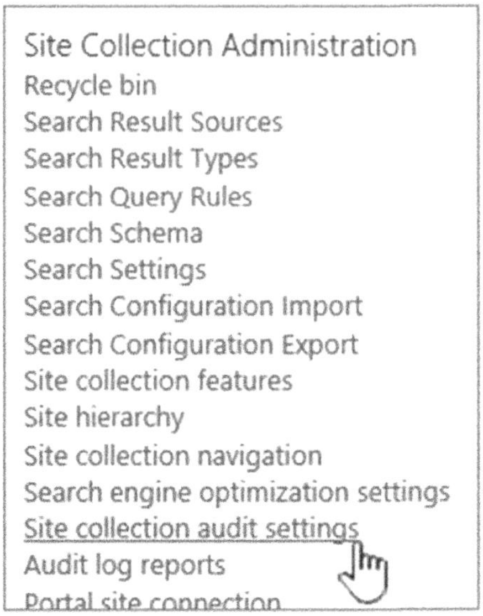

Figure 7-14. *Configure audit for site collection*

5. On the Configure Audit Settings page, in the "Documents and Items" and "List, Libraries, and Site" sections, select the events you want to audit and then click "OK."

Which events you audit depends on your auditing needs. For example, regulatory compliance usually has specific requirements that will dictate which events you need to audit. Additional unnecessary auditing can affect the performance and other aspects of your site collection(s).

Audit Reports

To view an audit log report, do the following:

1. Go to Settings ⚙ and then click "Site settings."

Note   The "Site Collection Administration" section will not be available if you do not have the necessary permissions, such as by being a member of the default Site Collections Administrators group.

---

2. Click "Audit log reports" in the "Site Collection Administration" section.

3. Select the report that you want, such as "Deletion" on the View Auditing Reports page.

4. Type a URL or browse to the library where you want to save the report and then click "OK."

5. On the Operation Completed Successfully page, select the "Click here to view this report" link. If you get an error, it may be because audit logs weren't enabled or there was no data to show.

    Notes:

    At least Excel 2013 must be installed to view audit log reports by clicking "Click here to view this report."

    Alternatively, if opening documents in the browser is enabled for the library, go to the library where you saved the audit log report, point to the audit log report, click the down arrow, and then click "View in Browser."

    You can use standard Excel features to narrow the reports to the information you want. Some ways in which you can analyze and view the log data include the following:

    - Filtering the audit log report for a specific site

    - Filtering the audit log report for a date range

    - Sorting the audit log report

- Determining who has updated content

- Determining which content has been deleted but not restored

- Viewing the changes to permissions on an item

The events that you select to audit are captured in audit reports that are based on Microsoft Excel 2013 and are available from the Auditing Reports page. You can also create a custom report that includes a number of these events over a specified date range, within a specific area of the site collection, or filtered to an individual user. You cannot modify events once they are logged, but site-collection administrators can delete items from the audit log and configure automatic trimming of the audit log data.

The audit log captures the following information for the events that are selected to be audited[1]:

- Site from which an event originated

- Item ID, type, name, and location

- User ID associated with the event

- Event type, date, time, and source

- Action taken on the item

Everything in this list can be automated, and you can write an elegant solution as well. One of the solutions written by the Microsoft folks can be found here: `https://github.com/SharePoint/PnP/tree/master/Samples/Core.ExternalSharing`.

Continuously Monitor Content Shared Externally

Once the site is created and a user starts using it, it will be essential for admins to continuously check what kind of sensitive data is stored in those external sharing sites and block those sites that are violating the data loss prevention policies.

DLP for SharePoint Online and OneDrive for Business is now built into the Office 365 Security & Compliance Center. It allows admins to search for sensitive content in the existing eDiscovery Center, keeping content in place and enabling the admin to search in real time, as shown in Figure 7-15.

---

[1]`https://support.office.com/en-us/article/Configure-audit-settings-for-a-site-collection-A9920C97-38C0-44F2-8BCB-4CF1E2AE22D2`

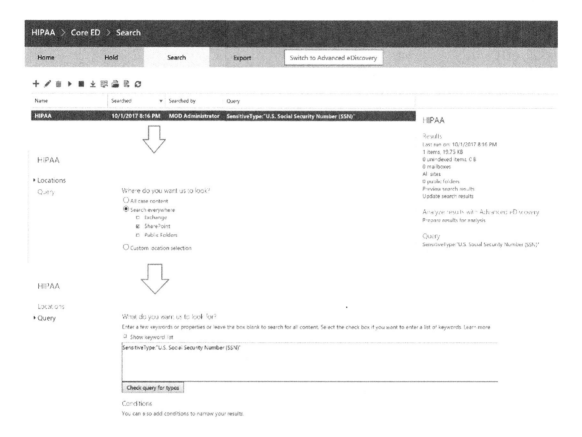

Figure 7-15. *Search files with sensitive content from eDiscovery Center*

The search results display sensitive content found in SharePoint Online and OneDrive for Business from within the eDiscovery Center in SharePoint Online, as shown in Figure 7-16.

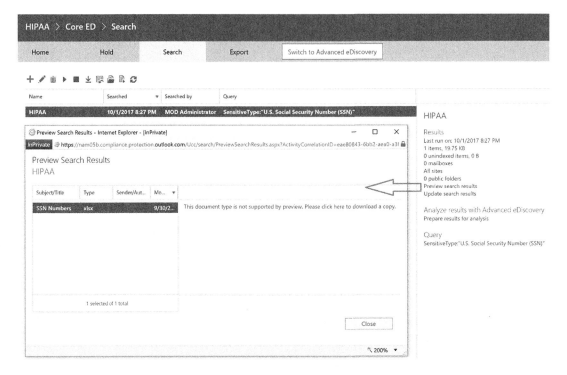

Figure 7-16. *eDiscovery Center search result for content with sensitive type in document*

Compliance officers can enter simple or complex queries and program Search to look at a variety of sources, including team sites and users' OneDrive for Business folders. Once the query is run, the results appear under the search result window, where the admin can review them in place. You can simply adjust the query, adding indexed properties such as "author" or "date" to fine-tune the results. It is important to note that permission to use the eDiscovery Center is role protected to ensure that the right people—not everyone in your organization—have access to run these queries and review sensitive content.

Adjust Policy Violated Documents

The admin will now be able to review possible offending documents inline, in real time—right from the eDiscovery Center. The admin will also be able to export the list of documents for further review and then take manual action, such as adjusting sharing permissions, removing data on shared sites, and more based on the review of the results.

Exporting the results is easy, and the admin can download a copy of the files with a report of the query results. The admin can save the query and then turn his or her attention to investigating the query results. The admin can inspect the documents, check for false positives, and further hone or expand the query if needed.

You can leverage the eDiscovery Center to find out if sensitive data is stored in those sites. See more at `https://support.office.com/en-us/article/Set-up-an-eDiscovery-Center-in-SharePoint-Online-A18F8975-AA7F-43B4-A7D6-001D14744D8E`.

Here are few PowerShell scripts to monitor the SharePoint Online environment:

```
Connect-SPOService -Url https://domain-admin.sharepoint.com
```

This command will get the list of all site collections where External Sharing is not disabled:

```
Get-SPOSite |Where-Object {$_.SharingCapability -ne "Disabled"}|select
Url,SharingCapability
```

This command will get you all the external users for a given site collection:

```
Get-SPOExternalUser -SiteUrl https://SPSite.sharepoint.com
```

This command shows you how to remove a user from the site collection:

```
$user = Get-SPOExternalUser -Filter TestUser1@contoso.com
Remove-SPOExternalUser -UniqueIDs @($user.UniqueId)
```

Conclusion

For any healthcare organization, it is very important to maintain data privacy in order to comply with regulations such as HIPAA and PII. As discussed in this chapter, organizations will have to make sure any data that is shared externally is completely secure and follows all regulatory standards. The administrator will have to prevent users from sharing documents externally from SharePoint Online and must establish an approval process for users who want to share documents externally. Administrators will also have to continuously monitor the site to make sure no confidential information is being leaked to the public. Securing documents with information rights management will provide an additional layer of security in case that document is leaked and accessed by users who do not have any right to open the file. Administrators or IT pros can extend the secure sharing capabilities via new tools like Power Apps, Forms, and Flow in Office 365.

CHAPTER 8

Continuous Education for Nurses

Healthcare and nursing are both currently riding a steeply cresting wave of change and innovation. It is difficult to point to any one event as the impetus to the change and innovation that has struck the healthcare industry in just the last few years. The book *Nine Shift* states that between 2000 and 2020, 75 percent of how we live our daily lives (work, life, and education) in the twenty-first century will change. Since we spend about 12 hours every day doing essential tasks such as eating and sleeping, for the rest of the 12 hours in a day, 75 percent, or 9 hours, will be spent doing things totally differently than we did just a few years ago. The last major shift was from 1900 to 1920, when we moved from an agrarian farming way of life to being industrialized, and now we are moving from an industrialized to a knowledge society. These predictions are already beginning to see fruition in many aspects of our lives, including healthcare and education.

Several recent historic events have catalyzed the nursing profession. In 2010, the passage of the Affordable Care Act represented the most extensive healthcare reform in the last 45 years, since Medicare and Medicaid. All parties—including legislative bodies, insurance agencies, healthcare agencies and providers, professional organizations, and potential patients—are immersed in transforming the healthcare system. With this comes a need for continuous education for nurses so they can stay up to date with new rules and regulations as well as to maintain their licenses.

Continuous education for nurses is mandatory in order to keep them current with their rapidly changing working environment. Nurses must complete ongoing education to keep their skills and licenses up to date or to enroll in courses in a new area of practice. Nurses also have to be educated about the environment they work in, like new hospital rooms, equipment, processes and rules, patient communication standards, and so on. Learning new skills and allocating time to do so is a challenge for many nurses. Healthcare organizations and local state boards make these trainings mandatory for

© Nidhish Dhru 2018
N. Dhru, *Office 365 for Healthcare Professionals*, https://doi.org/10.1007/978-1-4842-3549-2_8

their nurses to keep them actively engaged and employed as well as to maintain their licenses. Practicing nurses are often required to earn a certain number of continuous education units each year to maintain their licenses. Continuing education courses help them further develop their knowledge of a specific medical field. For instance, nurses may take courses on midwifery to increase their understanding of prenatal care. Other nurses will take courses to help them further their careers or prepare them to return to school to obtain a higher degree. The academic choices and desires of each nurse vary, and the applicable continuing education options are also varied. A few examples of such training courses are special healthcare problems; biological, physical, behavioral and social sciences; legal issues of healthcare; nursing administration; teaching of healthcare personnel and patients; personal development; registered nurse refreshers; clinical practice review, and so on. Nurses can even pursue an advanced degree in management, which is ideal for nurses who are interested in moving to a management position.

There are training institutes that provide different courses for nurses and keep the content current and relevant, for which they obviously charge hefty fees. This chapter will describe how by using existing tools and services, nurse managers or clinicians can make the training available to nurses cost-efficient. These trainings are all internal trainings for which videos are available to the healthcare providers. The team responsible for providing training uploads the videos to the video portal described next. There are instances where there are trainings that are very specific to local healthcare organizations and local rules and regulations and are shared with existing nurses to reinforce the message or with newly hired nurses to make them aware of local hospital rules, methods, and codes of conduct. This chapter will focus on this type of training and will showcase how to make such training available consistently irrespective of device and location.

Here are some reasons why healthcare providers might emphasize the importance of continuous education for nurses:

Advancement: To become a registered nurse (RN), entry-level nurses may take courses that help them in that direction. Registered nurses may take courses to learn about advanced practice opportunities, such as becoming clinical nurse specialists or nurse practitioners. Once nurses advance into these roles, they may take courses to continue to develop professionally, gain credentials, or even prepare them to enter doctor or nursing practice degree programs.

Maintaining Credentials: Healthcare organizations sometimes require that nurses continue their education even though they are practicing. Organizations such as the National Council of State Board of Nursing or the American Nurses Credentialing Center require nurses to take courses to maintain active licensing status.

Quicker Ramp-up Time: Healthcare organizations want nurses to be effective from day one and cannot afford to spend days training nurses by sending them to training institutions. On-the-job training via quick tutorials is the best way to familiarize the nurses with the environment and local policies.

Improving Patient Satisfaction: Highly trained nurses can increase patient satisfaction by approaching the patient in the right way and providing care in a more prescribed way. Patients also get similar care across all nurses, which results in fewer errors and repetitive questions answered by patients.

The US Bureau of Labor Statistics (BLS) reported an annual median salary of $67,490 for registered nurses in 2015. According to BLS projections, jobs for these professionals should increase by 16 percent, or faster than average, from 2014 to 2024. Continuous education is a way to maintain and develop nursing skills. An employer or licensing board may mandate a certain type or amount of ongoing education, or a nurse may choose to pursue it for professional development or to enhance future opportunities. Nursing is a rapidly growing field, with median salaries in the high $60,000s.[1]

Nurse Training Powered by Microsoft Stream

Continuous training is required not only for nurses but also for everyone who is providing care. This chapter will describe the nurse use case but is not limited to only nurse education. The following section will describe new tools for providing training with easy-to-use applications anytime, anywhere, using any device.

Microsoft Stream Overview

Microsoft Stream is an enterprise video service where people in your organization can upload, view, and share videos securely. You can share recordings of classes, meetings, presentations, training sessions, or other videos that aid your team's collaboration. Microsoft Stream also makes it easy to share comments on a video and tag timecodes in comments and descriptions to refer to specific points in a video and discuss with colleagues.

---

[1]"Nurse: Continuing Education Requirements for Nurses," http://study.com/articles/Nurse_Continuing_Education_Requirements_for_Nurses.html

Microsoft Stream is a secure video service, so you can manage who views your video content and determine how widely to share it within your organization. Secure application access is enabled by Azure Active Directory, a recognized leader in identity-management systems, to protect sensitive corporate content.

Microsoft Stream also helps you organize content into channels and groups so it's easier to find. Microsoft Stream works well with other Office 365 apps like Teams, SharePoint, OneNote, and Yammer, giving users even more ways to discover relevant content. Microsoft Stream tracks the total views of the video; however, if your organization needs to view who watched which video, then that functionality is currently not available in the Microsoft Steam service.

If you are using Office 365 Video and would like to transition to Microsoft Stream, see Transition from Office 365 Video.

Get started with Microsoft Stream in minutes and view videos on all your devices from anywhere, anytime. For more details on a particular topic, see the following sections.

Preparing for Training

Log in to the Office 365 portal (`https://portal.office.com`) using your work account. Click on the Stream icon on the main page (Figure 8-1).

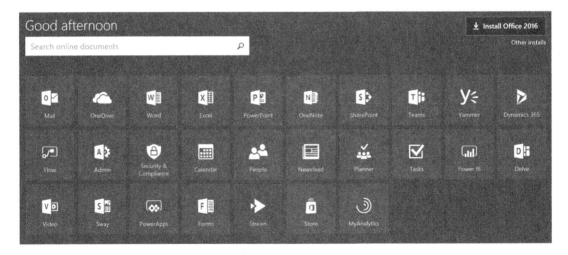

Figure 8-1. *Open Stream from Office 365 portal*

Groups in Microsoft Stream are a way both to organize videos and to control access to videos. You can define a set of owners and members of a group. Each group gets its own mini video portal, with a highlights page showing trending and new content within the group. Groups can be even further organized by creating channels within the group. Video can be uploaded into one or several groups to help viewers find it more easily. To create a group, click on Create ➤ Create Group from the top menu of the Microsoft Stream portal. As shown in Figure 8-2, a screen will pop up in which you enter information for creating a group.

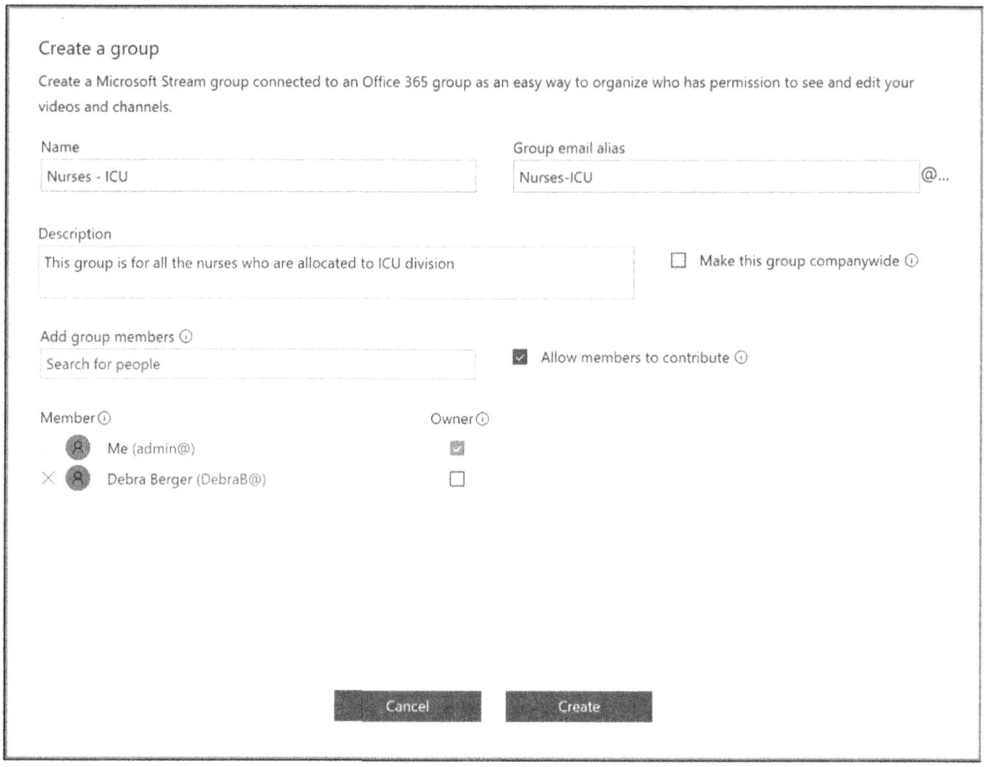

Figure 8-2. *Create Group in Microsoft Stream*

The group can be created companywide or for a specific group of people. Companywide groups give everyone in the organization access to upload and delete videos.

Microsoft Stream supports creating multiple channels that can be targeted to specific groups of people or specific topics. Channels don't have any permissions on their own but can be part of a group. Nurses and physicians can follow the channel and can get updates on new videos added to it. Each channel can contain one or many videos. Channels can be companywide, in which case anyone in the organization can add and remove videos, or they can be specific to a group. Figure 8-3 shows the Microsoft Stream portal homepage.

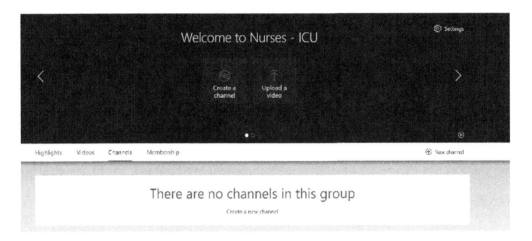

Figure 8-3. *Microsoft Stream portal homepage*

Figure 8-4 shows how to create a channel in Microsoft Stream.

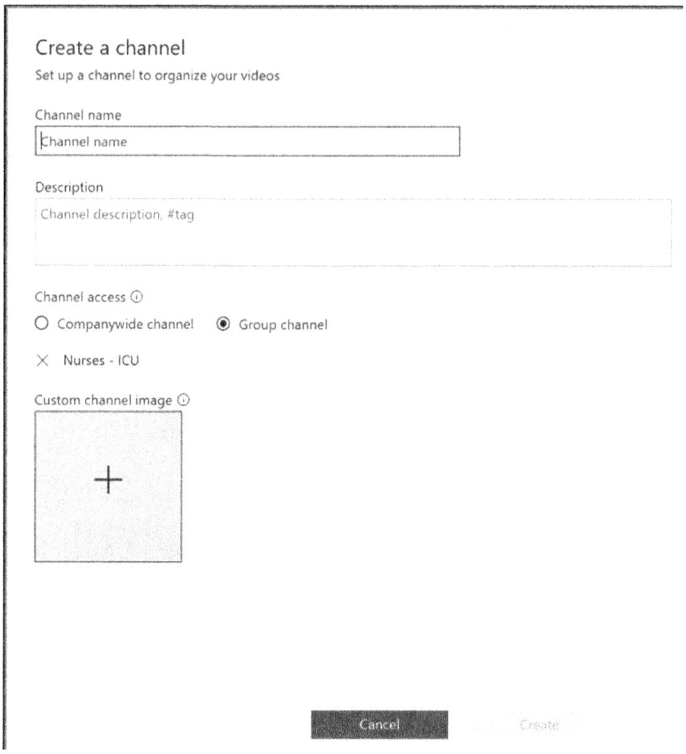

Figure 8-4. *Create channel in Microsoft Stream*

After you have created a channel, videos can be uploaded to the channel and consumed by the target audience. Figure 8-5 shows how the video will appear in the Microsoft Stream portal.

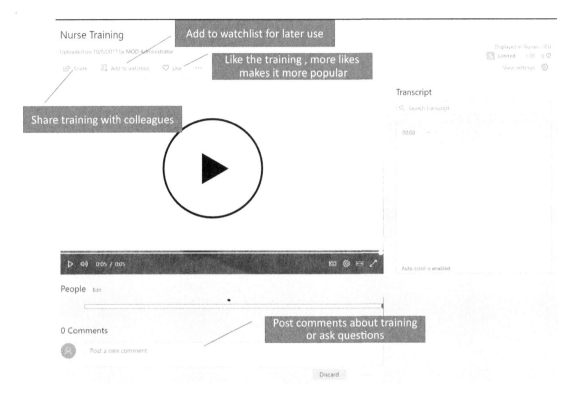

Figure 8-5. *Microsoft Stream video page*

Taking the Training

After the training videos are uploaded to the group or channel in the Microsoft Stream portal, links to those channels or groups can be sent out to participants for the training. Training videos can also be shared to a group of people or to the entire company via the Share ⬆ Share icon. There are also other ways to find the training, like searching for the training or from the popular or trending videos section.

To search for a training video, type a word or phrase into the *Search* box at the top of Microsoft Stream. Press Enter or click the magnifying glass as shown in Figure 8-6.

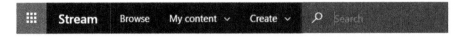

Figure 8-6. *Microsoft Stream menu*

This search is performed across all the channels, groups, and videos, or even within videos and their transcripts. Another way to view training videos is by following the channel. Once a user follows the channel, all the newly added videos within that channel will be automatically visible to them. Another method to view the training videos is through trending videos. The home page of the Stream portal features a few trending videos. Trending is determined by the number of views and the number of likes. Nurses or physicians can view all the trending videos on the homepage and can add them to their watch list to watch later.

Access Anywhere Using Any Device

Nurses and physicians can watch training videos using any device, such as PC, Mac, or mobile device. Navigate to a video by selecting a video thumbnail from the homepage or from the search/browse page, and the video will begin playing automatically in the browser window. The player controls can quickly and efficiently control the playback experience. Captions can be toggled on or off, playback speed can be changed, and the mode can be switched from regular to theater. Microsoft Stream supports various browsers for video viewing, such as the following:

- Edge for Windows 10
- IE 11 for Windows 10, 8.1, 7
- Chrome (latest) for Windows 10, Android (latest), Mac OS (latest)
- Safari (latest) for Android (latest), Mac OS (latest)

Nurse Training Powered by Teams

Chapter 5, "Innovations in Tumor Board Review," describes in detail how to configure MS Teams and its various channels. This section will focus on the nurse training use case and will assume that the reader knows how to configure and operate MS Teams. MS Teams can be used for creating a team of nurses or physicians and providing them the latest trainings. Microsoft Stream can also be integrated with MS Teams so that nurses and physicians don't have to leave the MS Teams interface to view the training videos. MS Teams gives nurses and physicians a way to make trainings more interactive. Nurses can ask questions in the MS Teams conversation section and can upload related files to the files section.

To add a Microsoft Stream training video to MS Teams, go to a team and click on plus to add a new tab, as shown in Figure 8-7.

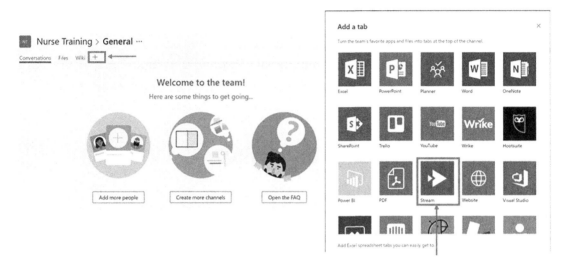

Figure 8-7. *Microsoft Teams interface for adding Stream channel*

Grab the URL of a video from Microsoft Stream and paste it in the screen shown in Figure 8-8.

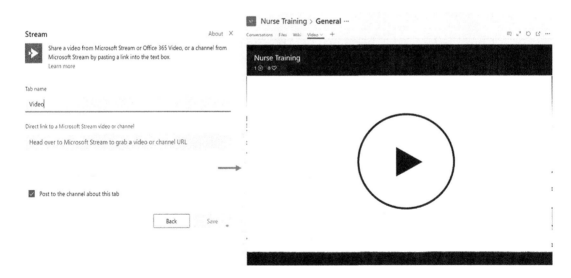

Figure 8-8. *Microsoft Stream in Microsoft Teams app*

This should show the training video from Microsoft Stream in MS Teams. Nurse collaboration has a positive impact on patient care because of the cross-pollinating clinical knowledge, and also because of the atmosphere that a collaborative spirit can yield. It tends to make the entire staff more at ease and attentive to patients, thus more effectively engaging with patients in their own care.

Broadcast Instructor-led Trainings

Nurses often attend workshops or conferences to stay current on nursing trends and improve patient care. Healthcare providers and nurse educators bring speakers from outside the hospital facility to educate nurses on current trends. Nurses travel for these trainings either to various healthcare facilities or to resorts or convention centers. Day-long workshops sponsored by hospitals often feature guest speakers who discuss ways to communicate better with patients and resolve nursing issues. These conferences and seminars sometimes qualify for continuous-education credits. These gatherings often focus on leadership and personal development or on a specific area of nursing, such as trauma, brain injuries, or strokes. Even though there are lot of benefits to participating in this type of training, it is also not possible to be at every conference and at every internal training because of work and personal commitments.

Technology can ease this pain by offering recorded sessions via virtual delivery on available devices; nurses can view the videos at their convenience. Office 365 provides call and video broadcasting features, which are good for virtual training. Skype Meeting Broadcast is a feature of Skype for Business Online and Office 365 that enables organizations to schedule, produce, and broadcast meetings or events to online audiences of up to 10,000 attendees. To enable this feature for your organization, do the following:

- Log in to `https://portal.office.com/adminportal/home` using your global administrator account.

- In the Office 365 Admin Center, go to Admin Centers ➤ Skype for Business.

- In the Skype for Business Admin Center ➤ Online meetings ➤ Broadcast meetings. Then, click "Enable Skype Meeting Broadcast," as shown in Figure 8-9.

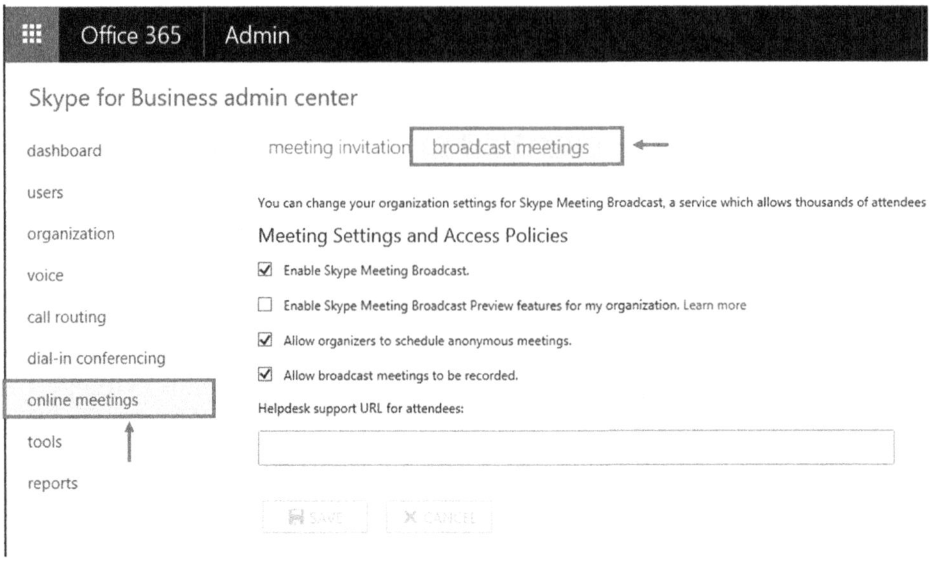

Office 365   Admin

Skype for Business admin center

dashboard

users

organization

voice

call routing

dial-in conferencing

online meetings

tools

reports

meeting invitation   broadcast meetings

You can change your organization settings for Skype Meeting Broadcast, a service which allows thousands of attendees

Meeting Settings and Access Policies

☑ Enable Skype Meeting Broadcast.

☐ Enable Skype Meeting Broadcast Preview features for my organization. Learn more

☑ Allow organizers to schedule anonymous meetings.

☑ Allow broadcast meetings to be recorded.

Helpdesk support URL for attendees:

💾 SAVE   ✕ CANCEL

Figure 8-9. *Office 365 portal inside Skype for Business Admin Center*

To schedule a meeting, browse to `https://portal.broadcast.skype.com` using your work account. Click on "New Meeting" and provide the needed attributes, as shown in Figure 8-10, to create a new meeting. Click on "Done" after providing all the attributes.

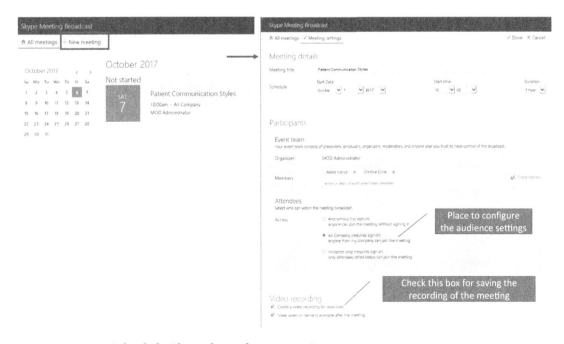

Figure 8-10. *Schedule Skype broadcast meeting*

After being scheduled, newly created meetings will show up on the meeting broadcast landing page.

The meeting scheduler can send an Outlook invite to all the participants by clicking on the meeting and opening the Outlook meeting invitation, as shown in Figure 8-11.

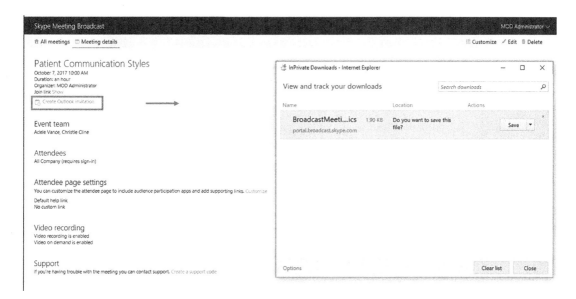

Figure 8-11. *Send Outlook invitation to participants*

Participants will get the email invitation once it is sent. At the scheduled time, they can click on the "Join the meeting" link to join the broadcast meeting, as shown in Figure 8-12.

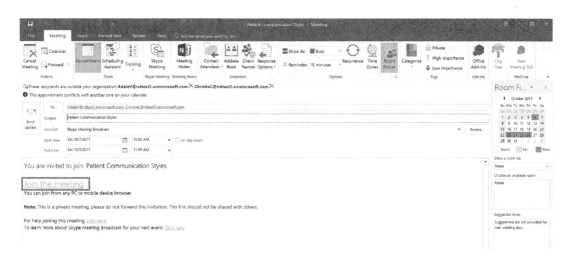

Figure 8-12. *Outlook invitation for Skype Meeting Broadcast*

After clicking "Join the meeting" either the Skype for Business client will open or the Skype for Business web application will open. Depending on whether there are video or voice calls, the Skype for Business interface will join the user to the conference as shown in Figure 8-13.

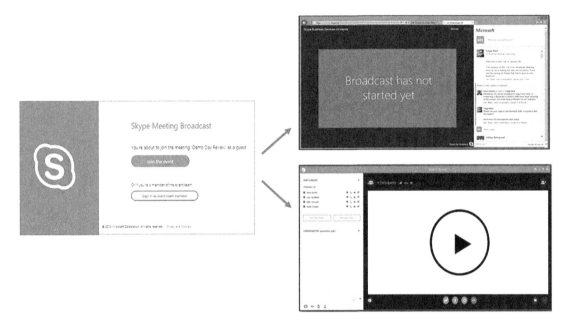

Figure 8-13. *Joining Skype Meeting Broadcast*

Skype Meeting Broadcast is a one-way communication meeting by default. In this meeting, participants are in listen-only mode. However, to make the meeting bidirectional, Skype Meeting Broadcast enables other interactive channels such as Microsoft Pulse, Q&A, and Yammer feeds. As shown in Figure 8-14, the meeting scheduler has the option to add these channels in the same window as Meeting Broadcast.

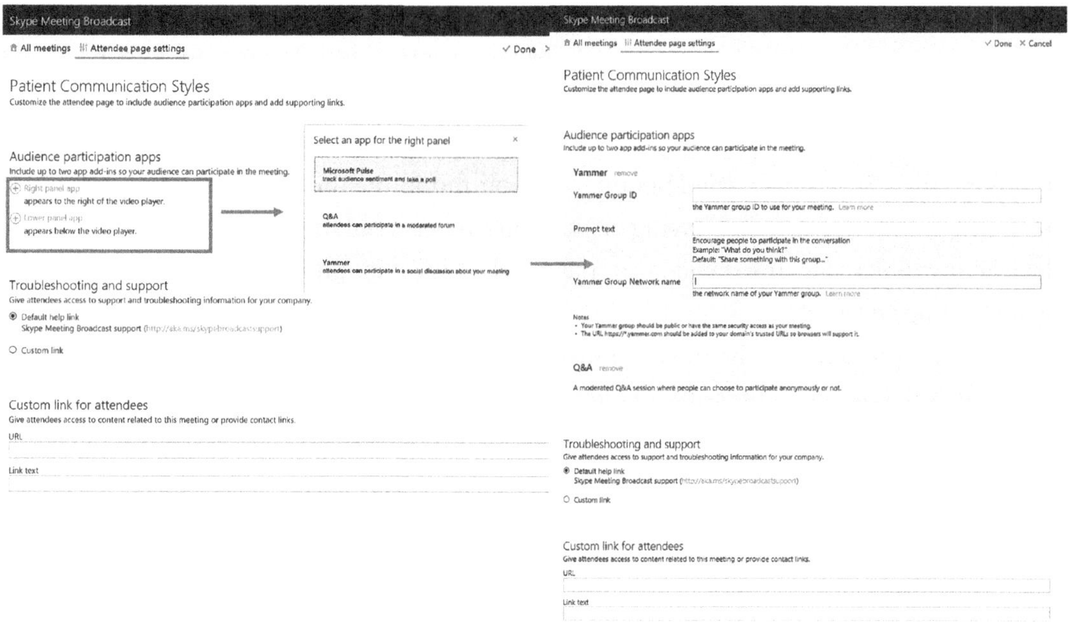

Figure 8-14. *Adding audience-participation apps*

Conclusion

Continuous education for nurses aims to create high-quality, patient-centered care in a healthcare system where nurses are essential partners in achieving success. Nursing across the globe is changing technologically, and nurses must be committed and willing to evolve and embrace inevitable change. Studies have long shown that morbidity and mortality statistics for hospital patients decrease as the educational level of the nurse increases. Some nursing employers are citing this data in their decisions to hire only better prepared and more highly educated nurses. The future is not far where online nursing programs with innovative teaching strategies will be needing to meet the needs of nurses across the county. Lifelong learning to prepare to take care of diverse populations throughout the lifespan can only be accomplished if continuous education is promoted and made mandatory for every nurse in every healthcare organization. Additional incentives should be offered to those nurses who are always up to date and willing to become a lifelong learner. The nurse educator role is going to be the key for this transformation in the healthcare delivery system. Nursing educators will have to incorporate more simulation and creative teaching techniques to improve clinical reasoning skills among nurses. Healthcare providers will have to think creatively to take trainings from brick-and-mortar locations to more simulation-based training where the latest tools—such as those mentioned in this chapter—will be used so that nurses can learn to interact with other healthcare professionals to coordinate patient care. It is predicted that as much as 25 percent of all clinical experiences will be available via simulation to provide a safe practice environment for nurses and healthcare professionals; this has the added benefit of accommodating the increasing enrollments in nursing across the nation.[2] Having virtual training be available to every nurse at any place at any time using any device will make nurses more competent and will remove the technology barriers.

These are just a few of the most significant drivers of nursing education today. Evaluating the impact on outcomes validates the importance of continuous education for the nursing profession and the value of nurses' contributions to inter-professional teams, and ultimately to the delivery of safe, high-quality patient care.

---

[2]Nursing Education Challenges, Carol Wilson, PhD, FNP-BC, RN, May 2011 - Volume 7 - Issue 11

CHAPTER 9

Monitoring and Lowering the Readmission Rate

Patient readmission, as defined by Medicare, is when a patient is admitted to a hospital within 30 days of being discharged from an earlier hospitalization, regardless of in which hospital the patient was originally hospitalized. Under the Hospital Readmission Reduction Program (HRRP), hospitals with readmission rates that exceed the national average are penalized by a reduction in payments across all their Medicare admissions— not just those which resulted in readmissions. There is no doubt that compared to the 1990s readmission rates have significantly come down in recent years. As a result of Medicare's readmissions reduction program, hospitals are working hard to bring the readmission rate down. Avoidable readmissions are a strong indicator of a fragmented healthcare system that too often leaves discharged patients confused about how to care for themselves at home and unable to follow instructions or get the necessary follow-up care. Medicare reports spending $17.8 billion a year on patients whose return trips to the hospital could have been avoided.[1] Readmissions are costly for a provider that doesn't have enough resources to spare, not to mention the 2 percent readmissions penalty stipulated by the Affordable Care Act.

By providing better care, providers can reduce the readmission rate, and, as a result, fewer patients will be revolving back through the hospital door. Providers have invested in care transition programs that reach beyond the hospital walls into the community. A tide of innovation aiming to improve care transitions out of hospitals is now sweeping through the hospital sector, largely motivated by Medicare's performance measurement. Healthcare providers and policymakers have noted that socioeconomic factors may often play a role in access to home and community support services that can aid a

---

[1] "Reducing Hospital Readmissions: It's About Improving Patient Care," *Health Affairs Blog*, August 16, 2013.

© Nidhish Dhru 2018
N. Dhru, *Office 365 for Healthcare Professionals*, https://doi.org/10.1007/978-1-4842-3549-2_9

patient's recovery after hospitalization. For example, lower-income communities and families may have limited resources for reliable transportation to take patients to follow-up medical appointments, assistance with patient mobility and daily living needs during recovery, and access to food that meets patients' special dietary needs. Further examination of ways to address patient and community needs in low-income areas may offer insights into ways to lower hospital readmissions in hospitals with a high share of low-income patients. Many studies show that hospitals can engage in several activities to lower their rate of readmissions, such as clarifying patient discharge instructions, coordinating with post–acute care providers and patients' primary care physicians, and reducing medical complications during patients' initial hospital stays.

Discharge Instructions and How-to Videos

Many patients are visual learners and can better retain information from videos than from reading patient handouts. Videos can also be interactive with Q&A sections and quizzes so that not only the patient but also their relatives can stay engaged, thus better supporting patients once they leave the hospital or staying educated while patients are at home. Video is one of the most powerful ways care providers and patients can connect, communicate, and learn as it breaks down geographic boundaries and brings a distinctly human element to digital interactions. Providers can leverage the Office 365 Stream service as a training vehicle for all the information needed either during their hospital stay or once they get back home. Patients can log in to the Stream service and view the training videos via any device from any location. Providers can record discharge instructions, including how to take care of themselves while home and what to do in an emergency, for patients at high risk for readmission, making it available online via the easy-to-use Office 365 Stream app. Office 365 Stream can also help with training and deploying community health workers to assist high-risk Medicaid patients with care transitions to reduce unplanned readmissions. The Office 365 Stream service can also track the patient views (as shown in Figure 9-1) so that providers can take action if patients are not viewing the training videos at regular intervals.

Microsoft Stream

Microsoft Stream is a sub-component of Office 365, or it can be accessed independently. Microsoft Stream lets care providers upload training videos or any other type of video into the platform with a very easy drag-and-drop function. Nurse managers or case managers can upload relevant videos into their own channels to segregate the content and target it to the right audience. Microsoft Stream is built on top of the recommendation engine that surfaces content based on relevance via machine-learning capabilities. Providers do not have to store large video files in their on-premises storage locations or worry about spending an enormous amount buying more storage. Microsoft Stream will let patients view training videos using any device from any location. This will increase the reach of the videos to more patients, as now there is no barrier to getting to those videos, even if the patient is in a remote place. Microsoft Stream will also make sure only authorized patients have access to the videos, and only those who have collaboration rights will be able to upload videos to the platform.

A nurse manager or case manager will start by creating a channel in Microsoft Stream. Once the channel is created, videos can be uploaded to the channel. This is a good way to organize the videos into different categories, so patients can get to them without any confusion. Figure 9-1 shows the "Patient Training" channel and the few videos uploaded to it.

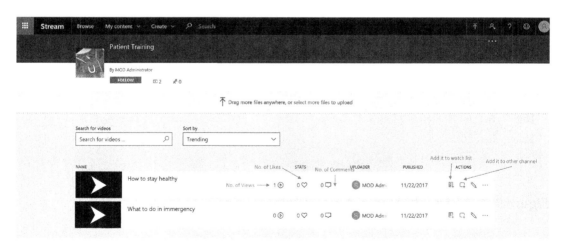

Figure 9-1. *Microsoft Stream channel page*

Microsoft Stream has analytics built into it, as just shown. The number of views, likes, and comments are tracked per video and per user level. The same video can be made available for more than one channel. Patients can create their own personal watch list based on topics they are interested in. The admin can assign videos to specific channels and then assign patients to it so that the patient is not lost in a system filled with videos. Admins can also limit access to channels by creating a group channel. In this channel, admins can specify a group of users who will have access to the channel; otherwise, users will not be able to view the videos in that channel. Figure 9-2 shows how to create a group channel.

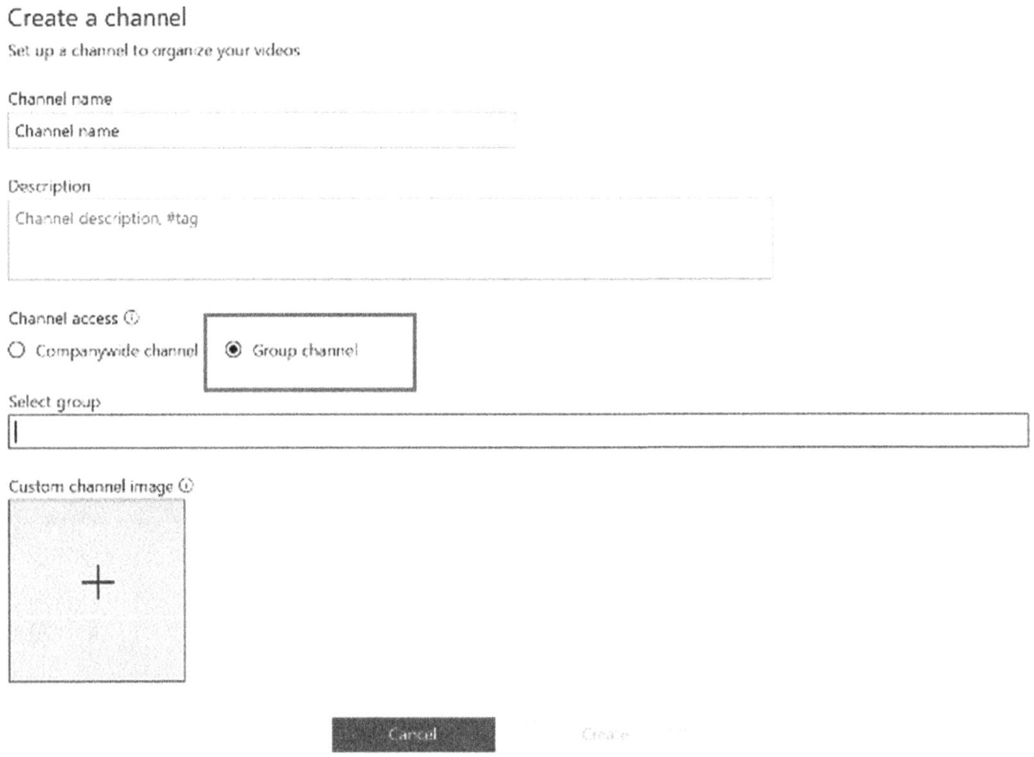

Figure 9-2. *Microsoft Stream channel-creation page*

The admin can create a group inside Microsoft Stream and keep it either private or public. That is the group that will be displayed in the preceding screen. The following process shows how to create a group within Microsoft Stream:

1. Click on Create ➤ Create Group from the top banner of the Microsoft Stream portal.

2. Provide information required to create a group, as shown in Figure 9-3.

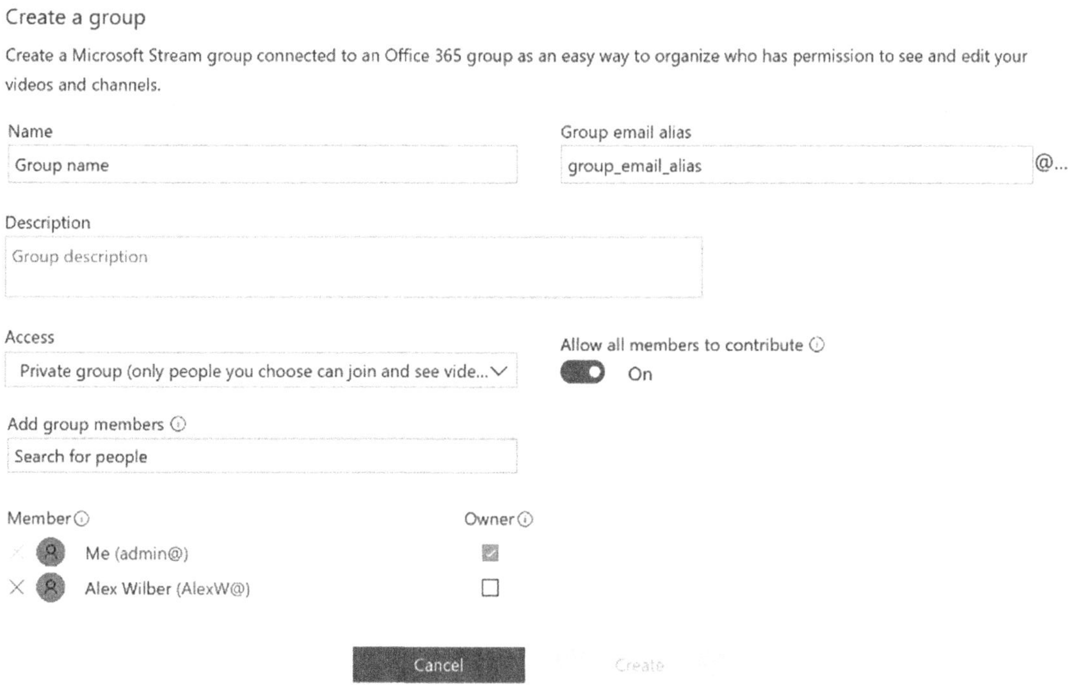

Create a group

Create a Microsoft Stream group connected to an Office 365 group as an easy way to organize who has permission to see and edit your videos and channels.

Name

Group name

Group email alias

group_email_alias   @...

Description

Group description

Access

Private group (only people you choose can join and see vide... ∨

Allow all members to contribute ⓘ

⬤ On

Add group members ⓘ

Search for people

Member ⓘ

× Ⓡ Me (admin@)

× Ⓡ Alex Wilber (AlexW@)

Owner ⓘ

☑

☐

Cancel   Create

Figure 9-3. *Microsoft Stream group-creation page*

3. Click on "Create" to create the new group.

Following a Schedule

Discharging patients from the hospital is a complex process that is fraught with challenges. There are over 35 million hospital discharges annually in the United States. Premature discharge or discharge to an environment that is not capable of meeting the patient's medical needs may result in hospital readmission. There are several approaches to improving the discharge process, as follows:

- Pre-discharge interventions: This category includes activities such as patient education, discharge planning, medication reconciliation, and scheduling a follow-up appointment.

- Post-discharge interventions: This category includes activities such as follow-up phone calls, communication with ambulatory provider, and home visits.

- Bridging interventions: This category includes activities such as transition coaches, patient-centered discharge instructions, and clinician continuity between inpatient and outpatient settings.

The healthcare team must determine the most appropriate setting for ongoing care when it has been determined that a patient is medically ready for discharge. To determine the most suitable discharge plan, the provider should involve patient, family, case manager, nurse, physician, physical and occupational therapists, social worker, insurer, and so on. After considering all these parties and their various needs, the provider prepares a care-continuum plan, which the patient must follow after going home or to another care facility. The patient should be able to access this plan anytime and should be able to track the progress. Paper-based care plans are difficult to maintain, easy to lose, and lack real-time updates for the provider on the patient's progress. This is where newer technology like Office 365 Planner helps. The following section will describe how Planner can be used in patient discharge planning.

Office 365 Planner

Office 365 Planner makes it easy for the care team to create new plans, organize and assign tasks, share files, chat about questions or concerns, and get updates on health progress. Office 365 Planner is another tool for providers outside of the main Electronic Health Record (EHR) system, so if providers do not want to maintain separate tools then Office 365 Planner might not be a good tool for them. Office 365 Planner could be a good tool if the provider wants to take the conversation and planning outside of the EHR system, such as a nurse's non-patient-related task assignments or a nurse manager planning tool. The provider can decide after going through the following section whether this is of interest, as Office 365 Planner comes with the Office 365 subscription at no extra charge.[2]

One of the most valuable aspects of Planner is that it helps care teams organize the patient schedule visually. Each plan has its own Board, and within each Board, each work item or task is represented by a Card that can have due dates, attachments, categories, and conversations associated with it. Patients receive an email notification whenever they are assigned a new Card or added to a conversation, as shown in Figure 9-4.

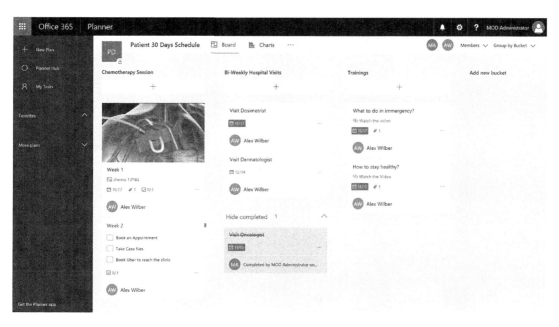

Figure 9-4. *Planner home page*

The patient will see the dashboard when he/she goes to Planner portal or app. Each Board (Chemotherapy Session and Bi-Weekly Hospital Visits from the figure) shows the list of tasks the patient must complete before the due date. Each task can have several properties, such as title, assigned to, start date, due date, status, description, attachments, checklist, comments, and so on. The case manager can take ownership of creating and maintaining a schedule in Planner. Every time a new task is assigned

---

[2]https://blogs.office.com/en-us/2015/09/22/introducing-office-365-planner/

under the Board, the patient gets notified via email. Every Card can have documents (or pictures) attached that automatically get rich image previews, so it is easy to understand what the Card is about at a glance. In addition, Cards can be organized on the Board into customizable columns called Buckets, which can be prioritized and tagged with colored labels, as shown in Figure 9-5.

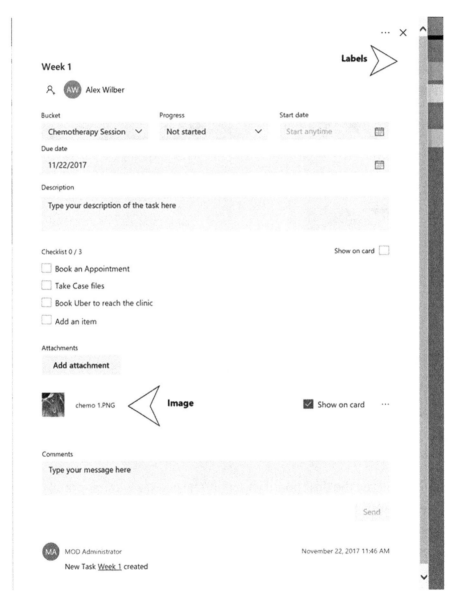

Figure 9-5. *Planner new task creation page*

Planner also offers views to keep the patient-care schedule on track. The Hub view lets patient and provider track overall progress across all plans, while the My Tasks view lets the patient filter down to see just what he/she needs to do across every plan. In addition, the Charts view includes interactive charts for visualizing the patient's progress against deadlines. The patient can click a red segment on the histogram to quickly see which aspects of a plan are behind schedule. With Planner, everyone on the care team is always on the same page. A single glance at the Charts view, as shown in Figure 9-6, is all it takes to know where things stand for the care providers.

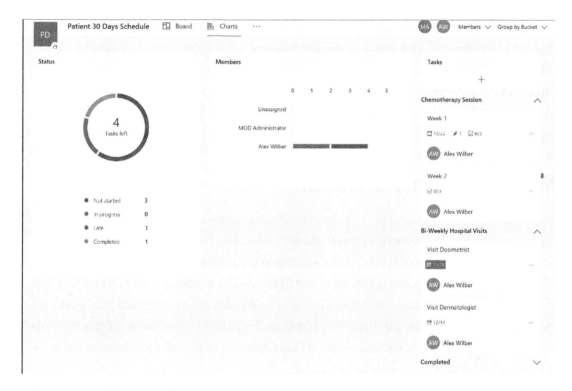

Figure 9-6. *Planner Chart view page*

As shown in this figure, the patient gets a graphical representation of all the tasks that are completed, pending/late, or upcoming/not started. The patient can easily click on any of those tasks and take appropriate action.

Patients can also use mobile phones or tablets to update their tasks on the go. Patients can update their tasks status and view their next task, and the app will always keep them updated on what is pending via email notifications.

Discharge Summary

A recent study by J Hosp Med. 2016 Jun;11(6):393-400. Epub 2016 Feb 23 shows that a delay in completion of the discharge summary was associated with higher rates of readmission. Around 87,994 patients were studied for their discharge summary between January 1, 2013, and December 31, 2014, and the conclusion was that more days taken to complete discharge summaries was associated with higher rates of all-cause hospital readmissions. Timely discharge-summary completion time may be a quality indicator by which to evaluate current practice and is a potential strategy to improve patient outcomes. Even though the discharge summary is crucial to lowering the readmission rate, unfortunately the discharge summary reaches the primary-care provider by the time of the first follow-up visit in only 12 to 34 percent of such visits, and even then it often lacks key information.[3] Computerization of the discharge summary is needed for faster exchange between hospitals and primary-care providers and to maintain a continuous patient history.

Microsoft Planner Notebook

Microsoft Planner can be used to update the discharge summary in the same Planner page that the case manager has prepared for the patient. The same caveat applies as in the earlier introduction section; this is going to be a separate system outside of the EHR system and is not a replacement of the EHR system, so use this tool as needed. The nurse manager can update the entire discharge summary in the notebook and make it available in the same Planner page that contains the patient schedule information. That way, all the patient discharge information is available in the same tool. To attach the notebook to Planner, follow these steps:

1. Go to the patient's Planner page and click on "Notebook," as shown in Figure 9-7.

---

[3]Kripalani, S., LeFevre, F., Phillips, C.O., Williams, M.V., Basaviah, P., and Baker, D.W. "Deficits in communication and information transfer between hospital-based and primary care physicians: implications for patient safety and continuity of care," JAMA. 2007 Feb 28;297(8):831-41. Review. (https://www.ncbi.nlm.nih.gov/pubmed?term=17327525&report=docsum)

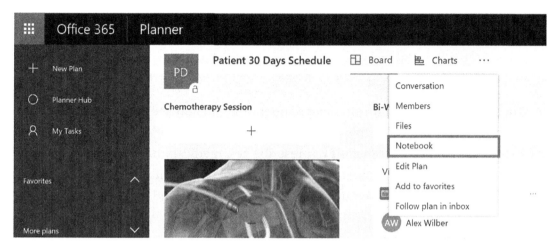

Figure 9-7. *Create Planner notebook*

2. New browser windows will open with a notebook where all the information can be noted, as shown in Figure 9-8.

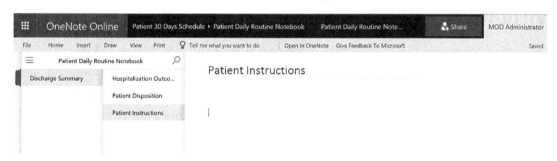

Figure 9-8. *Planner notebook view*

3. The notebook can have several pages and sections for various information, as shown in Figure 9-9.

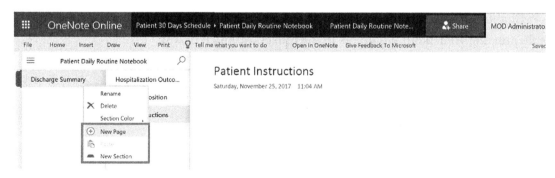

Figure 9-9. *Create a new page or section in Planner notebook*

"New Page" will create a new page inside the current section, which is "Discharge Summary" in the preceding screen. "New Section" will create a new section parallel to the existing section "Discharge Summary."

The patient's primary-care physicians and nurses can now see the discharge summary and schedule using the same tool. Based on the patient's condition, physicians can modify the medication schedule or prescribe new medication. Physicians can also write new notes inside the Planner notebook to update the hospital that new medication has been prescribed to meet certain conditions. Hospital staff and primary-care provider staff now have one holistic view of everything related to when the patient is discharged from the hospital and ongoing treatment with local care providers. This helps significantly to reduce the communication gap between hospitals and primary-care providers, which in turn helps reduce the readmission rate.

Virtual Visit by Nurses

Once the patient is at their home after discharge, nurses can follow up via Skype calls on a regular basis, ensuring medications and discharge instructions are being followed and patients are attending follow-up appointments with primary-care physicians. Nurses don't have to spend long hours traveling to a patient's home, but instead can use that time to virtually meet more patients and help them with their care coordination. Once the Planner is set as per the preceding section, nurses can check the tasks' status and follow up via Skype call first, and if the patient is not reachable, then they make a visit to the patient's home. Status updates in Planner can also be automatically updated based on smart medical devices, assuming those devices can interact with API-based systems that Planner supports.

Chapter 4 has more information on virtual visits via skype and how telehealth can help providers reach more patients in the most cost-efficient way.

Conclusion

Managing readmissions is a complex task, but thanks to the Medicare program, hospitals are taking an important leadership role that was previously unfilled. With technological innovations and a willingness to try them out, providers will bring down the readmission rate even further. It is important to understand how care management provides improved clinical outcomes for patients and improved satisfaction for providers. The primary-care doctor always has the challenge of looking after their patient post–hospital discharge, especially with conditions such as coronary artery disease post–bypass surgery, end-stage renal disease, and diabetes, which can be complicated by near blindness.

Because the Hospital Readmission Reduction Program (HRRP) affects Medicare payments to hospitals, its effect on Medicare patients is generally indirect. To the extent that the financial penalties encourage hospitals to implement activities designed to improve care quality and lower their rate of preventable readmissions, the penalty program could be beneficial to Medicare patients and the Medicare program. Alternatively, some have noted that reducing financial resources to lower-performing hospitals could have a negative impact on their delivery of patient care. Regarding beneficiaries' out-of-pocket expenses, a hospital's penalty status has no direct effect on beneficiaries' cost-sharing during inpatient stays. For readmissions, the inpatient hospital deductible ($1,316 in 2017) is waived, but beneficiaries do face other out-of-pocket liabilities—mostly in the form of coinsurance for separately billed physician services received during their stay—as they would in all inpatient stays.[4]

---

[4]Cristina Boccuti and Giselle Casillas, March 10, 2017, "Aiming for Fewer Hospital U-turns: The Medicare Hospital Readmission Reduction Program," (`https://www.kff.org/medicare/issue-brief/aiming-for-fewer-hospital-u-turns-the-medicare-hospital-readmission-reduction-program/`)

Index

A

Ability MyCite, 4
Active Directory Authentication Library (ADAL), 32
Active Directory Federation Services (ADFS), 29–30
Advanced Encryption Standard (AES), 46
Advanced Threat Protection (ATP), 14, 24–25, 37
Affordable Care Act, 173
American Telemedicine Association (ATA), 75
Audit settings configuration
  audit reports, 167–168
  events to audit, 165–166
Azure Active Directory (AAD), 16
Azure Active Directory Connect (AAD Connect), 28
Azure Information Protection (AIP), 58, 64

B

Business associate agreement (BAA), 55

C

Cloud identity, 16
Common Security Framework (CSF), 61
Continuous education, nurses, 173

broadcast instructor-led trainings, 183–187
importance, 174
training by Microsoft Stream, 175
  access anywhere, devices, 181
  overview, 175–176
  preparation, 176–177, 179
  taking training, 180–181
training by MS Teams, 181, 183
training institutes, 174

D

Data loss prevention (DLP)
  policy, 22–23, 37–38
  configure HIPAA, 156
  creation, 155
  EOP, 57–58
  GDPR, 64
  protect sensitive information, 153–154
  rules configuration, 158
  target sharepoint/onedrive accounts, 157
  user notification, 159
  violation icon, 160
Data privacy, 69
Delve Analytics, 11
Digital pill, 4
Digital technology, 53

© Nidhish Dhru 2018
N. Dhru, *Office 365 for Healthcare Professionals*, https://doi.org/10.1007/978-1-4842-3549-2

Get the eBook for only $5!

Why limit yourself?

With most of our titles available in both PDF and ePUB format, you can access your content wherever and however you wish—on your PC, phone, tablet, or reader.

Since you've purchased this print book, we are happy to offer you the eBook for just $5.

To learn more, go to http://www.apress.com/companion or contact support@apress.com.

Apress®

Printed in the United States
By Bookmasters